The names and identifying characteristics of some of the individuals featured throughout this book have been changed to protect their privacy.

HarperCollins books may be purchased for educational, business, or sales promotional use. For information, please email the Special Markets Department at SPsales@harpercollins.com.

First HarperOne hardcover published 2021

FIRST EDITION

Designed by Leah Carlson-Stanisic

Library of Congress Cataloging-in-Publication Data
Names: Tsabary, Shefali, 1972- author.
Title: A radical awakening / Dr. Shefali Tsabary.
Description: First edition. | San Francisco :
HarperOne, 2021 | Includes index.
Identifiers: LCCN 2020051622 (print) | LCCN 2020051623 (ebook)
| ISBN 9780062985897 (hardcover) | ISBN 9780062985903
(trade paperback) | ISBN 9780062985910 (ebook)
Subjects: LCSH: Self-realization in women.
| Self-actualization (Psychology) in women.
Classification: LCC HQ1206 .T79 2021 (print)
| LCC HQ1206 (ebook) | DDC 155.3/33—dc23
LC record available at https://lccn.loc.gov/2020051622
LC ebook record available at https://lccn.loc.gov/2020051623

21 22 23 24 25   LSC   10 9 8 7 6 5 4 3 2

A
RADICAL
AWAKENING

Turn Pain into Power,
Embrace Your Truth, Live Free

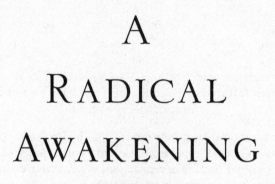

DR. SHEFALI

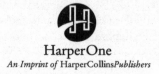

HarperOne
An Imprint of HarperCollins*Publishers*

A
Radical
Awakening

Every radical awakening needs a spark.
This spark ignites the eternal self.
Without that, none of this.

This book is an ode to one of the deepest
friendships I have known.

With another and with myself.

Contents

Infinite gratitude to my brilliant editor, David Ord, who has stood by my side through every book I have written.

Also, to my amazing editor at HarperCollins, Gideon Weil, who believed in this project right from the start.

And to my daughter, Maia, who inspires me with her authenticity on a daily basis.

Thank you for holding my hand through this process.

The Time of the Awakened Woman

There comes a time in the life of a woman
When she discards her old ways like tossed shoes in the garbage
When she shreds her list of "shoulds" and obligations
And when impossible expectations are burned in an incinerator

There comes a time in the life of a woman
When the approval of others once jewels now turn to pennies in
    her sock
When the hunt for another is now replaced by a hunt for herself
And when parental tentacles of tradition no longer define her truth

There comes a time in the life of a woman
When her desire to fit in with the crowd dissolves
When her manic compulsion to be perfect vaporizes
And when her obsession to be voted popular eviscerates

There comes a time in the life of a woman
When she simply says "no more"
When facade, artifice, and guile leave her nauseated
And when righteousness, dogma, and superiority repulse her

There comes a time in the life of a woman
When she no longer fears conflict but faces it boldly like a lioness
When she guards her authenticity as fearlessly as she guards her
    babies
And when she drops the role of savior knowing she can only save
    herself

There comes a time in the life of a woman
When she no longer cowers in the shadows of her unworthiness
When she no longer plays small so others can feel big
And when she swaps the role of victim for the role of cocreator

There comes a time in the life of a woman
When she unabashedly and boldly occupies her ultimate sovereignty
When she finally feels ready to claim her space in the world
And when she redefines compassion as unequivocal self-love

There comes a time in the life of a woman
When she finally releases her childlike dependencies on others
When she dares to rewrite a new mandate of living for herself
One that says:

    I release unworthiness and fear
    I divorce servility and passivity
    I divest inauthenticity and enmeshment
    I end the pretense of being someone I am not

    And from now on I declare . . .

    I will ascend into my highest power
    I will embrace my greatest autonomy
    I will celebrate my deepest worth
    I will embody my fiercest courage
    and manifest the most authentic me

    The time is now
    I am ready
    To awaken into my renaissance.

A Love Note to My Sisters
Before You Begin This Book

This book is about your awakening. It is an ode and an homage to your authentic self, the self that is waiting to be birthed anew.

We all yearn to be free, yet we feel encaged in our daily lives, consumed by fear and unworthiness. What these pages promise you is a path out of the cage toward a new vision of yourself.

To awaken and evolve means to deeply understand ourselves. This involves befriending the parts of us we may not want to see, especially our pain. When we fully accept our pain for what it is—without sugarcoating it, and certainly without apologizing for it—and observe the many ways we have cocreated it, we can begin to transform the pain into wisdom.

Understanding our pain is painful. This is why the words on these pages may trigger you. I want you to know that I have been intentional with these triggers. They are meant to ignite and evoke an inner revolution. The pain comes from a dismantling of old belief structures and ways of being. The feelings of shock, grief, and loss are therefore not only natural, they are pivotal for your transformation. You may not realize it, but you are capable of the evolution I advocate. More than this, you are worthy of it. Here, I share my own experiences so that you know you are not alone. I have walked in your shoes in my own way. Because of this, I understand how challenging this journey called life can be.

I gently forewarn you that this book is going to pack a punch, especially at first. Put on your emotional seat belt before getting on this ride. Because this book is an exposé of all the ways we have been asleep, it isn't a comfortable read. When we shift into a new awareness, we tend to go through a severe disorientation. You will be provoked in unexpected ways and may want to put the book down at many points during this journey. We all have a natural resistance to the harsh truth awakening brings.

Be assured that just by picking up this book you have embarked on the first critical step of your quest for authenticity. The structure of the book echoes the pathway of your psychological and spiritual unfolding. As such, your journey is already underway.

Allow for insight to wash over you. Take your time as you read. Pause, reflect, journal. Let these pages be the birthing canal that lead to your authentic emergence.

So let's begin, sister. We've got this. Let's enter the ocean together. There is a new horizon on the other side. It's called freedom.

Disclaimer

While I have tried to include as many human experiences as I could, it is possible I may have left many out. While I also mostly speak of the male-female relationship, I try, in some cases, to include all ranges of sexual orientations.

My intention is to be as inclusive as possible. I fully honor that the human experience manifests in infinite ways and that each is worthy of equal dignity. If you find yourself feeling excluded, my suggestion is to not get too focused on the exact manifestation of external behavior, but instead on the internal dynamics to which I allude.

In the tapestry of our inner experiences, we have more in common than we realize. Here you will find resonance and, through it, a path toward your own evolution.

A
RADICAL
AWAKENING

Part One

~

ASLEEP

in the

MATRIX

~

Soul Erosion

Like a sword in a sheath, her brilliance stays dormant

Like a bow in a quiver, her power stays invisible

Like a pea in a pod, her worth stays small

Like a trapped animal in a cage,
she awaits permission to be freed

Like a butterfly in formation,
she will only emerge when her old skin dies.

I knew I was in trouble when I found myself in a ditch on the side of the road with zero recollection of how I got there. I had fallen asleep at the wheel and my car had stopped inches from a tree. Exhausted from mothering my toddler and coping with a rigorous PhD program in tandem, without any help from relatives or nannies, I had burnt myself to the ground. The jolt woke me up. I could barely breathe and my entire body was shaking. Jittery and confused, I was luckily able to get my car back onto the highway. Thankfully, there was no injury to anyone. Even my vehicle was undamaged.

The incident brought to the fore another kind of casualty that had been eroding me from within for a long time—the serious destruction I had been doing to my *soul*.

Soul erosion is a gradual process—a slow, creeping, chipping away of our inner being, resulting in the inevitable death of all we know to be our truest selves. It's a disease that begins in childhood and spreads contagiously, especially in women. Its symptoms include loss of power, authenticity, voice, and vision. Soul erosion is essentially an obliteration of our inner knowing. Each incident in which we suppress our inner truth, we engage in the erosion of our most precious treasure—our essence.

Let me illustrate how this happens. Trista, one of my clients, remembers being around four years old when she broke her favorite toy—a doll she had named after herself and took care of like it was her little baby. Heartbroken, she recalls crying for hours. Her father, a strict disciplinarian, told her to stop crying or else she would get a spanking. This made her cry even more.

When she continued crying at the dinner table, her father lost his temper, broke the rest of her doll, and dumped it in the garbage. Shocked by his rage, Trista recalls being stupefied. "It was like he had broken me into pieces and dumped me in the garbage. I wanted to cry and scream. I actually wanted to hit him and break him, but instead I just stood there, frozen. No one came to my rescue. No one comforted me. For the first time I realized what it meant to be abandoned. He didn't just throw my precious doll away, he discarded my entire sense of safety, security, and worth. I could never trust him or my mother in the same way again." From that moment, it dawned on her that she needed to hide her true self. This is how her lifetime armor of emotional stoicism formed.

To this day, even in her forties, Trista has a challenging time expressing her inner world and feelings articulately. Both her husband and children often complain to her that they don't feel connected to her because she is too harsh and rigid. Her teenage son, Matt, in particular had been entering into almost daily conflicts with her, which led her to seek therapy with me. It was only after much processing that she came to understand how her childhood defenses—emotional withdrawal and suppression—were now interfering with her ability to connect with her son.

Trista was repeating her childhood pattern to the letter, even personifying some of her father's old ways. When Matt expressed his feelings, Trista found herself being critical and harsh with him. Now she understood why. He reminded her of her younger self, the one who was reprimanded by her father. When she saw him being emotional, she interpreted it as weakness and sought to squash his feelings, invalidating him just as she had been. As she brought her old memories into awareness, she began to heal the wounds of her old self and, in this way, opened her heart to her son.

At first, our true self fights for survival. It protests loudly, so much so that we feel nauseated. As we continue to ignore it, the protesting fades until it's a mere whimper. As the years erase all memory of its existence, the plaintive cries recede altogether.

This loss of self is universal. We have all felt its ravaging wounds. As our authenticity erodes, what's left behind is a cavernous inner crater filled with a cacophony of chaos that infects every part of how we now live. It manifests in all sorts of insidious and seemingly insignificant ways:

Cars careening off roads
Alcoholic blackouts
Eating disorders
Chronic exhaustion
Self-doubt and sabotage
Purposeless jobs
Missed deadlines
Forgotten bills
Listlessness and apathy
Confusion and self-loathing
Emotional disconnection and withdrawal
Gnawing anger and irritability, and so much more

My near-death accident shook me into the awareness that not only had I veered off the road, I had veered off my soul's reason for being here. Who was I? Who had I become in the flurry of gaining my PhD, while trying to be a wife and a mother? How had I allowed my essence to be destroyed and discarded in this way?

I was so good at hiding my inner life that no one would know I was emotionally disjointed and falling apart. My veneer of competence was brilliantly put together, covering my internal disarray and misalignment. I wore a mask of supercompetence and achieve-ment. After all, I had been creating this outer persona for decades and it was now well honed.

As it is with all of us, the death of who we originally are is re-placed by a persona we commonly call the *ego*, our false self. Most of us grow up thinking of this as our *true* self. Little do we realize that we are creating an entire life based on a false foundation that will have severe emotional consequences for years to come.

The Role of the Ego

The birthplace of the ego is self-abnegation. It thrives when the in-ner self is ignored, denied, suppressed, and all but annihilated in favor of a force on the outside—typically the voice of others, espe-cially our loved ones, the culture in which we are raised, or a sys-tem of beliefs that captures our imagination.

There isn't a person I know who has escaped the replacement of their authentic self with a persona, the mask behind which their true self lies largely dormant. This happens more so with little girls because of the overarching patriarchy we live under, where boys are allowed to "just be boys." Our young girls, on the other hand, are trained to fit a rigid prescription early in life.

So conditioned are women to abandon any vestige of inner truth for the sake of fitting into what our parents or culture want for us that we go through life unaware such a split even exists. Sometimes we may feel a rumbling within that shows up as discontent or in flares of anger, but we downplay these as a "mood" or attribute them to some issue that ruffled our feathers. We bypass our inner schism unaware that it is creating deep crevices in our lives.

Most of us grow into adults unaware of the false ways we have ad-opted in order to get our needs for love and worth met. If we happen to be shaken awake, as I was when my car left the road, we typically run for cover, before long recycling our old way of being. Things stay much the same under the guise of "good enough."

With this in mind, you may be surprised to hear that the facade we refer to as the *ego* is actually a "good guy." The ego is a picture we carry of ourselves in our head, a way of seeing ourselves that meshes well with what our family and society expect of us. Having developed slowly in response to our upbringing, it cleverly teaches us a way of functioning that suits our everyday reality.

As children, we were unable to self-advocate. Growing up, we had no option but to surrender to the conditioning we received even if this meant a divorce from our essence. By creating a false self, the ego is, in fact, acting compassionately. As a necessary aspect of what it takes to grow up, the false self is something we instinctively adopt in order to ensure our needs get met. The tricky thing about the ego is that its coup of who we really are in essence is so gradual that we aren't aware of how it's changing us to fit in with our family and culture. Moldable as children are, we capitulate to our parents' dictates, often without pushback. We contort ourselves until we match the picture others have of us such that *their* picture of us becomes our *own* picture.

If our parents admonished us for being too emotional or too this or too that, many of us immediately reacted to their injunctions in some rapid-fire way, adjusting our temperaments to match their standards. As happened with Trista, the ego becomes our armor, our protector, helping us adjust to a misaligned childhood.

So great is our thirst to be seen and validated by our parents and our culture that we succumb to the ego's powerful and instinctive lure, slowly burying our authentic nature in the process. The result is a false identity, which we now present to the world. We think it's who we are, but it's really only a facade we wear to ward off the fear that we are unworthy and unlovable.

In the Fog

I can honestly say that I lived in a fog for much of my life. There were glimpses of my authentic self here and there, of course, but there were large parts of myself that stayed submerged for decades. Looking back at who I used to be, I cannot help but wonder how, when I felt emotionally invalidated or subjugated, I simply silenced myself. The woman I am today would never allow that to happen. Yet this same woman not only allowed it in the past, she rationalized it as her only choice.

This is what I mean by "being in a fog." The fog is an atmosphere that surrounds us, whether we are women or men. This fog produces vision blindness and results in a denial of reality. We don't see things as they actually are. This atmosphere is created by what we know as the *patriarchy*. This system of male domination brings with it an implicit silencing and denigration of women and children. The male who is accustomed to being at the top of the totem pole exerts his power over others to maintain command. This hierarchy has the potential to turn toxic when left unchecked. Referred to as *toxic masculinity*, it becomes the ambient cultural tone, leaving its emotional scars on both women and men. Quite simply, it "fogs" our lens of consciousness causing severe dysfunction in our lives.

As a result, women and children live in a subconscious state of wariness around men. We grow up knowing men are in charge. With this comes the awareness that there is a potential threat when we are around them. Every female instinctively knows to turn away from a group of men in an alley. This instinct isn't mere paranoia. It is an inner caution honed by strong cultural evidence of innumerable violations against us. Although protective, it is a burden that is heavy to bear.

Can you imagine how this awareness of a potential threat shapes our psyche? Whether we had a father who simply raised his voice occasionally or one who indulged in mad rages, we learn to instinctively protect ourselves around the males in our lives. This takes a toll on us and fundamentally shapes how we develop.

The patriarchy trains young girls to be like sheep following the herd. We are the original lost sheep, searching for our shepherds who, we are told, are either God, our father, or our future husband.

Like any flock, we follow well. We know the key ingredient of a good sheep is the ability to lose our unique identity, blend into the crowd, and become servile and passive. To shine out is unacceptable and against the rules of the flock. Being modest and dimming ourselves so that we fit in is essential. We learn early to disappear, becoming so invisible that we merge with the fog surrounding us.

I see many women who constantly make excuses for our ill treatment at the hands of the modern-day patriarchy. Our habit, *our automatic default,* is to think something is our fault, just as a child believes it's their fault when they receive a parent's neglect or ill treatment. This is why many of us don't call out toxic treatment. We don't even believe it's an option. So part and parcel of our daily experience is bad treatment, as we watch our mothers and sisters endure it all around us, we grow up believing this is simply the way things are.

This book challenges us to push against the status quo. It dares us to go beyond "how things are" to enter a new vision of ourselves. It begins by awakening us to our reality—how our biology shapes us, how our psychology molds us, and how our culture scares us until we lose ourselves. By understanding and embracing these three layers, we allow ourselves to break free.

The first step begins in calling the fog a *fog,* distinguishing it from reality. In my own life, it took decades to actually name what I was going through. I so lived in fear of the disapproval of others that in order to keep the harmony, I took on the blame for what I was enduring. If anyone behaved badly, it was because of something I did. I thought this was how I was supposed to take responsibility. Little did I know that all I was doing was deflecting the *other* from taking responsibility. By my taking the blame, the other could stay comfortable and, therefore, happy with me.

It took me a long time to realize the difference between taking on blame versus taking on responsibility. Whereas blaming myself kept me mired in fear, accompanied by my silence and complicity, taking responsibility allowed me to see my participation in my own victimization and rise up with courage and daring.

Fear is the ruling emotion in our fogged-up state. Because we live in fear, we don't call out the toxicity for what it is. Fear is followed by blame, topped off by shame for feeling such fears and not taking action against them. I saw this cycle of fear-blame-shame in my own life. Each time I didn't stand up for myself out of fear, I beat myself up for days afterward. It was only when I could own my fear that I began to awaken.

There are two arrows, you see? One is the actual denigration and silence we women endure. The second is the blame-shame we feel for having endured it. Deep down, we know we should speak up fearlessly. Our fear revolves around the following:

What will people say?
Who will I be without external approval?
Will speaking up affect me financially?
Will my children be okay?
Will I face emotional or physical harm?

Not only do we stay afraid, we can't help feeling nauseated by our lack of courage. Cycling between these fears keeps our own internal subjugation alive and kicking. Eventually we realize that we have to name it to tame it. We become ready to shout from the rooftops, "Me Too!" Instead of drowning in victimhood, we end what kept us in such a subjugated state.

I understand when women are pissed off, outraged, frustrated. They have suppressed their feelings for so long that it makes sense when they bubble over and feel the need to scream, "No more!" Such women are often labeled "irrational," "emotional," and "off the rails." They are likely to be socially ostracized. Scared that this might happen to us, we tend to avoid becoming so bold. Little do we realize that becoming a bold woman is our path to salvation.

As long as fear eclipses the language of our soul, we continue to be puppets to external forces. Under the tutelage of fear, our ego performs like an automaton. Robotically reactive, we become a slave to fear in its many forms:

Fear of rejection
Fear of failure
Fear of ostracism
Fear of loneliness
Fear of unworthiness
Fear of emotional or physical abuse

So conditioned are we to be afraid, we wear fear like a second skin. So pervasive is fear in our life experiences, we often fail to fully appreciate just how ruled by it we are. Because of our place in the patriarchy, we women allow ourselves to be silenced and bullied for fear of punishment by the often more powerful males in our life. Over time, this silent cowering becomes our internal default. It's often so subtle, we can barely discern it ourselves.

Whether we are in a toxic relationship or not, or have been physically abused or not, the fact is we are a hairsbreadth away from this possibility. Don't be fooled into thinking you're smarter or wiser just because you haven't fallen prey to an aspect of our patriarchy in a direct way. It's actually unavoidable. If you are a woman in today's world, you have felt it in some way or other. You may not recognize these experiences for what they actually were yet, but they happened and, trust me, they had an impact. There isn't a woman I know who has escaped the crushing weight of the patriarchy in which we live.

It took me years into my journey to accept how much I had allowed my own worth and voice to be crushed by the men around me. I'm almost ashamed to admit that I was so blind and conditioned as to allow myself to be silenced in the ways I did most of my life. I almost don't want you to know this side of me. I want you to project an aura of perfection, wisdom, and power onto me. Yet I also know that it's only when I lay bare the honest truth about my own awakening process that you may be able to begin yours.

It's always so much easier to hide our vulnerable sides, the parts of us that aren't so wise, so bold, or so "put together." Yet I know now that it's only when women share their processes—their true processes, the bare bones of them—that other women can feel safe to share theirs. It's in this sharing that we can collectively rise.

Leaning into the discomfort of revealing parts of ourselves we don't want to acknowledge, and certainly don't want others to see, is a crucial part of our healing journey. Unless we stare at ourselves and acknowledge all our inner parts, we will not enter wholeness. To integrate ourselves means to accept all of who we are—the done and *un*done, the kind and *un*kind, the strong and *not* strong. Wholeness doesn't mean perfection. It means acceptance—a raw and unabashed acceptance of exactly who we are in any given moment.

Sharing my life story in these pages has been an act of leaning into discomfort. At times, I resisted it out of fear of your disapproval, yet I knew that I had to work through these fears. If I didn't, I wouldn't share. And if I didn't share, I wouldn't grow. If I didn't grow, neither would you.

This discomfort is not only natural, it's the only way we shed the familiar and enter the new. We have been conditioned to run from discomfort. Yet I wish for these pages to show you that it's only when we run *toward* these shadowy places within ourselves that we will find our redemption, truth, and freedom.

Hitting Rock Bottom

I know I'm not alone on this quest for my true self. I've talked with thousands of women who want to get out of the fog and live more awakened lives. So oblivious are we that we are living from a false sense of ourselves—fear-ridden and suppressed—that it often requires multiple awakenings for us to face up to the fact.

I think back to my client Pam. She called me after a particularly harrowing day. She had spent the entire day tending to her family. She went through a litany of things she'd done for each of them: her elderly mother needed to be driven to the doctor, her ailing sister needed her home care help arranged, her daughter needed help moving furniture in her apartment, her youngest son needed help with homework, her husband needed her input on a project he was working on. Loving and kind, Pam thought that putting their needs before her own was what she was supposed to do. She had done this all her life and kept playing this self-sacrificing role. What Pam wasn't in touch with was the emotional toll it was having on her. She wasn't connecting the dots.

She had put on twenty-seven pounds in the last year. She and her husband had come close to divorce after she discovered his infidelity. She regularly lost her temper with her children. Instead of being in touch with her true feelings, she kept covering them up through the role she was desperately holding on to, believing it would deliver her the emotional salvation she craved. She was acting out her conditioned concepts of the kind of mother, wife, and daughter she believed she needed to be in order to be validated. And it was killing her. She just didn't know it. She was completely submerged in the fog.

When I gently suggested she was playing the role of rescuer and fixer in order to get her needs met, she retorted indignantly, "Are you suggesting I want to do this?" She could hardly believe I would imply such a thing. "Why would I do that?" she insisted. "Why would I willingly exhaust myself like this? Am I just a sucker for punishment?"

It took us a while to deconstruct her patterns so she could finally see how she had been playing the roles of fixer, giver, and rescuer without even realizing it. Pam had always been the savior in her family—the solution finder, the nurse, the mediator, the peacemaker. Where there was a need, she was the provider. This is how she had acquired her parents' love as a child. Whenever others in her life had a need, instead of allowing them to take care of themselves, she rushed to the rescue. When it came to loving another or receiving love, this was the only method she knew. It's quite possible she even attracted needy people so she could play out her familiar role. Over time, not knowing how to take care of herself through proper boundaries, she reached a breaking point.

Women are trained by culture to receive love through sacrificing ourselves. Such self-sacrifice takes on a myriad of appearances. Regardless of what they are, we believe that, through their embodiment, we will receive the love we desperately seek from our immediate families. This behavior slowly branches out to our friends and others. If our self-sacrificing roles keep bringing us attention—and it doesn't really matter whether this attention is positive or negative—we adopt them. Soon we cannot tell if the roles are even roles or if they are our true selves. Little by little, just like Pam, we begin to melt down, either through exhaustion or as a result of a crisis. Our veneer cracks and light begins to enter through tiny crevices.

The arrival of light where there was only shadow before feels traumatic. As we are stripped of our roles for the first time, perhaps, we feel bereft on one hand and strangely alive on the other. These feelings are so shocking, our instinct is to cover the crevices back up with old patterns and forget what we glimpsed. However, over time and with enough trauma, the crevices enlarge. The ego can no longer cover up the cracks. When this happens, we frequently refer to it as a "breakdown." If it occurs later in life, we call it a "midlife crisis."

Typically, only excessive trauma can shake the ego off its axis. When this happens, we may hit rock bottom. As a therapist, rock bottom is the experience I wait for in a client. It signifies the potential death of the ego. Whereas the client avoids it desperately, trying every which way to bypass its final reckoning, the therapist waits for it with bated breath. At rock bottom, the real self is forced to strip off its mask, often leaving the person feeling like a stranger to themselves. There is a sense that nothing works anymore. All our tried-and-true strategies that we use to run from the truth of who we are now seem to fail.

The day my car swerved off the road was my rock bottom. It was at that moment I realized I needed to make changes right away. I didn't know where to begin or how. All I knew was that it was time. My soul could stand to be eroded no further.

When we reach rock bottom, the silent denigration we allow at the hands of culture or our parents must be fully acknowledged and repaired. The hard part is seeing this "allowing" part of ourselves naked in the mirror. It's almost too unbearable to accept that we have let ourselves be torridly neglected and belittled.

What now? Should we go back to being who we were raised to be? Can we really return to living in a fog—a cloudy haze of fear, rituals, traditions, and conveyor-belt predictability?

If we are truly at rock bottom, the choice is often made for us. We can keep pretending it isn't, but it is. Our minds can make up all sorts of fantasies, tricking us into believing that everything is the same as before. But deep down, we know we are avoiding the stark truth.

The reason why rock bottom hurts so much is because our ego's facade has cracked under pressure. Our usual habits and strategies no longer work: they have bottomed out. We now feel emotionally bereft. This new place feels scary and threatening. Who are we without our usual egoic defenses?

If only we realized that hitting rock bottom and undergoing the cracking of our ego is the portal to our rebirth, we wouldn't dread it so much. Because we don't trust this is all happening for our own betterment, we resist. This is understandable.

Without our childhood scripts and patterns, and minus culture's impositions, who are we? Have we ever examined who we might be when stripped of our facade? If we are courageous enough to see the answer, we are on track to find the true purpose of our lives—to be our most authentic self in the here and now. This means digging deep into our essence and shedding all that isn't true to who we are. It means releasing the parts of our being that no longer serve us and letting go of patterns that keep us stuck. It means looking squarely at our fear of doing so and confronting what lies behind it.

For Pam, it meant shedding her need to be validated as a rescuer and fixer. As she increasingly validated her inner self, she released those around her from giving her that ego fix. As she grew to love herself more, she began to say no more often. At first, those close to her resisted her new way of being and even felt betrayed by her, which is a normal reaction. When they realized they had no choice, they began falling into line.

Pam had let the light in. She had finally tasted what it meant to be free of the script that she needed to sacrifice herself in order to receive another's validation. She was able to answer the question all of us arrive at on our path toward spiritual awakening: "Am I ready to be true to myself, and give myself the validation I so desperately sought from others until now?"

From Fear to Love

How did we learn to stay silent in the face of fear? It's like we instinctively knew from childhood that it was wiser to remain silent than to protest. When I got groped on the bus, cat-called on the street, harassed in the store, or straight up abused by this man or that, I learned to swallow my dignity. I was always afraid to face retribution if I made too much noise. I was more attached to how others saw me than I was to being authentic. Every abused woman will attest to this. We all stay quiet because we're afraid that speaking up will cause others to disapprove of us, making things worse.

Cultural oppression and subjugation are the masters of our psyche, and fear is the curriculum they mete out on a daily basis. We are graded on how silent and subservient we are. The more quiet, the higher the grade. These are the legacies of a patriarchal culture that has everyone messed up, including men. Such is the nature of a toxic system. It doesn't spare anyone from its clutches.

When we enter fear and its offspring silence, we move away from self-love. One of the hallmarks of self-love is the honor and free expression of our inner worlds without blame or shame. Constant suppression of our authentic voice creates a gnawing and growing inner disconnect. By pushing away and ignoring our authentic experiences, we promote the illusion they didn't even occur. This dissociation provides fleeting comfort, but over time it causes us to lose touch with our moment-by-moment experiences. The greater the dissociation, the greater the lack of inner connection and alignment. Soon, what we say, think, and do are grossly out of touch, leaving us feeling anxious and bereft.

When we give into culture's manipulation, playing safe and playing small, the patriarchy stays in power. The antidote to culture's suppression is a daring rebellion against silence. There is no nobility in suppressing and abnegating our voice. Such oppression doesn't do anyone any good. It simply encourages and upholds the dominance of the patriarchy.

In most of the adult intimate relationships I've had with men, I stayed in fear. Bold and daring in my career, I was the opposite in my personal interactions. I was inauthentic and allowed myself to fade into oblivion. It took me years to fully awaken. One denigration after another, one suppression after another, one more moment of denying my inner truth was slowly building up pressure. I pretended nothing was going on, until one day I couldn't anymore. Then everything blew to smithereens.

I can write this book on radical awakening because I have walked the path of hot coals myself. I lived so many years being false to myself that I understand what it takes to get out of the fog. My goal is not to focus on the pain as much as to show women it's possible to transform pain into power.

We don't want to see how burying our truth is an act of war against ourselves, but it very much is. Unless we recognize this, we will keep doing it to ourselves. When we allow toxicity to exist for the sake of peace, we are actually perpetuating war. There is no real peace where there is no authenticity. Lasting peace only emerges from an honest acceptance of oneself and one's life experiences.

Self-love blossoms when we claim our experiences through our expression and our actions. Each time we honor our feelings and inner process, we declare self-love. When we rebel against culture's embargo against our voice, we give ourselves and each other the space to be heard and seen.

Imagine if women everywhere began to speak their authentic

truth about how it really feels to be who they are, including their fears and failures. Can you imagine the release of pressure we would feel? We would no longer need to walk around feeling cloistered and suffocated, pretending to live perfect lives. We would set ourselves, and each other, free.

When a woman tells the daring truth of what she has endured, she moves away from being mired in individual fear toward a new emotion—love. She declares, "I love myself. I am worthy of being heard. I am more than the sum of my past. I trust my voice."

In this book, I challenge women to shift from fear to love. When we tell our stories and feel witnessed, we experience an integration within ourselves. Soon there is a growing coherence and a growing wholeness within us that might not have been there before. When one woman manifests the courage to speak up for herself, like a tidal wave, she clears the path for other women to empower and emancipate themselves. When she begins to live in authenticity, others are emboldened to do the same. The focus shifts from fear for her own well-being to love for all. She understands that by ending her own fear, she is actually loving herself, her sisters, and her daughters.

As we begin to notice how we participate in our own self-suppression, we can take small steps toward self-expression. It may take time because we are unaccustomed to hearing ourselves speak our truth. We can begin with a close friend or a maternal figure, perhaps. Or we can enter coaching or therapy to work with a relative stranger. As we do so, we consciously manifest who we truly are, rather than being unconscious and passive victims.

Awareness of how culture has suppressed and silenced us allows us to understand our psyche better. This awareness is not passive. It requires careful scrutiny of our internal dynamics and how they have been set up by our conditioning. Through this active process of deconstruction and discernment, awareness moves into awakening.

As you read these words, you may feel intimidated or overwhelmed. You may feel inadequate in some way. If you do, I am

here to assuage those emotions by telling you that there is no perfect way to awaken. It is not about getting to a destination either. It
is, quite simply, just about your unfolding—an unfolding that will
occur naturally as you allow these words to enter you. This is the
way of consciousness. It is akin to light bulbs getting turned on in
an otherwise dark room. These words are your light bulbs. As they
turn on, you will begin to see what was previously in the shadows.
Once the light is on, you cannot help but see. It is a natural outcome
of your new consciousness.

You are here. This is huge. Let's take a deep breath and move on
to the next chapter together.

2

The Idea of *That Woman*

You cannot just be good, only great

Not great, only greater

Not greater, only excellent

Not excellent, only perfect

Not perfect, only a war against the self.

Whenever I get into a relationship, I lose myself," women frequently tell me. It doesn't surprise me when women inform me they are in a relationship that's destroying the last shard of who they once were. It doesn't surprise me because, through the inner work we will do together, I know they will come to realize that their relationship isn't where the destruction of their authentic self began. The relationship is just evidence of the final collapse of an already shattered inner world.

No one loses themselves to another. They come to the other *already lost.*

Straying from ourselves began decades before we became an adult and entered a relationship. The proclivity to wander far from our true self essentially got drummed into us with our mother's heartbeat while we were in her womb. The way we find ourselves today came down the generational pike, we just don't realize it until a relationship begins to mirror our lostness. If we are lucky, we see the pattern and wake up.

While it isn't something we are consciously aware of, most women are trained from early girlhood to crave what I call the triple threat: the need for *approval, validation,* and *praise.* This triple threat is a means of glossing over the void that lies at our center, where our essence was intended to blossom. Lacking awareness of who we truly are, the triple threat becomes our unconscious surrogate—a sort of aphrodisiac.

When I speak of our *essence,* I'm talking about an identity that's moored at the core of the self. This vision of ourselves is untethered to any external goal. When we have the space and exploration to roam free, firmly planting ourselves in our own essence, we discover how truly powerful we are. The problem is that others have played the central role in our psyche more than we ourselves have. This is at the root of our sickness. The extent to which we are carved and curated by others is shocking.

Having worked with hundreds of women back home in India and here in the West, I don't believe I have met a single woman who wasn't raised to relate to others in this pliable, if not subservient, way. I'm not talking about being beaten and abused. I'm referring to an intense and radical confusion about who we are at our core. I am speaking of our common tendency to obliterate our identity for the sake of what others and culture demand of us. Regardless of the facade we wear, each woman battles a loss of her essential self at the hands of others. Who are we when stripped of our cultural conditioning, free of our identification as someone's daughter, sister, wife, or mother?

It's extremely important to understand our blueprint as women. No matter our geographical location or our income, or whether we were raised on a farm in Pakistan or Ohio, we were, to varying extents, formed by this blueprint. One may have received these foundational elements over a communal meal of goat biryani, the other over an after-church lunch of beef and potatoes. However they were passed on, in whatever language, the fact remains that we women are conditioned to hold ourselves back and give of ourselves to ensure that the needs of others, especially men, are met before our own. As a result, we often suffer exhaustion and burn out. We find ourselves irritable and cranky with little awareness of why.

It's from understanding how our self-abnegation or self-loathing came to be that the deepest self-love eventually emerges. To do this, we need to go deep within ourselves and understand the severity of our divorce from our inner being. Only then will our transformation flourish.

Part of the awakening process requires that we hold up a mirror to see every belief we falsely hold and every dysfunctional pattern in which we addictively participate. Until this painstaking and detailed audit of our inner workings is conducted, we will not spot our patterns and won't be able to break free from them.

The truth is that no one likes to see themselves as having been molded by culture and, even less, do we relish hearing that most of what we have believed about our role as women is a lie. It requires a long look within, where we dissect layer upon layer of conditioning, to discover the degree to which we have been hoodwinked. Since most of what we believe has been a lie, this is scary. What a shocking truth!

If you are experiencing reactivity around this, I understand. I get it. It was extremely hard for me to wake up to these truths myself. I felt betrayed by my parents and my culture. I was angry and frustrated. I wanted to shut down and withdraw from the world. These are natural feelings. Leaving the matrix is never a comfortable path. It is riddled with confusing emotions. However, if you can invite the discomfort in, as opposed to resisting it, you may begin to see the importance of this kind of detailed inner scrutiny.

The more we look behind our psychological cobwebs to understand what lies there, the less the risk that we will be ensnared by these webs in the future. But if we aren't even aware of how these webs hooked us, how will we keep from becoming entangled over and over again?

As hard as this inner work is, it also promises the greatest gift to you—the gift of authenticity. Most of us are unaware of how powerful a force authenticity can be in our lives. In my own life, it was only through the arduous, yet glorious, work of discarding my inauthentic layers that I began to touch upon my inner liberation.

This is what these words are leading you toward as well. I know they may rankle you at times and cause discomfort. I am with you, by your side, championing you. Let's keep going.

Is "Good" Really Good?

Although it manifests in different ways, most women subjugate themselves as a result of a common internal pressure, which can be seen in the question, *Am I good enough?*

Who on this planet can meet the standards posed by culture? You are correct—no one. But this is not what we are told. We are given the misguided sense that we can somehow—if we were just *this* enough or just *that* enough—miraculously become that good. This, of course, is a trap that leads to a gnawing and perpetual sense of unworthiness.

To value ourselves, love ourselves, and honor ourselves only if we are *x*, *y*, or *z* is the subconscious script we have been burdened with for too long. We treat ourselves as worthy only if certain criteria are met. We need to become someone or something, and only then can we achieve acceptance.

So pervasive is inauthenticity and loss of self that sometimes I think it's an aspect of a woman's emotional DNA. We seem to be conditioned to be lost, trained early to forget our true self, brainwashed to forfeit who we really are. We have been losing ourselves since before we were born, through our ancestors, generation after generation.

You may not identify yourself as lost, since lostness disguises itself in clever ways. It shows up in the following:

Fear in expressing one's voice
Inability to create healthy boundaries
Apathy and withdrawal
Irritable and impatient outbursts
Lack of sexual desire
Giving up of one's goals

Lack of self-care
Aimless busyness
Overwhelm and feeling torn
Confusion and ambivalence
Procrastination and self-sabotage
Insecurity and self-doubt
Ceaseless worry and anxiety
Addiction to food and substances

In order to obtain the three valuable drugs of *approval, validation,* and *praise,* women essentially shape-shift, morphing into whoever those around us wish us to be. After all, we are just being the self-abnegating individuals we were conditioned to be. This is especially the case if a woman grew up thinking of herself as "the good girl." "The good girl" tries desperately to be validated, seeking a sense of belonging and endorsement from her outer world. She learns early that her goodness comes from two main sources: *compliance* and *service to others.* Some who are raised as trophy children can add another motive to the list: *excellence.* This way of being forms an emotional template—a habitual way of responding to the outer world. Women then confuse this programmed way of being with their own true self.

There is a huge difference between being authentic and being good. We get so wrapped up in the messaging around being good that we completely forsake authenticity and alignment with our core being. Only when we begin to see how this attachment to goodness keeps us divorced from our inner knowing does our situation change.

But isn't it good to be "good"?

If only it were so simple. The problem is that good is only a benign sounding cover-up for something far more sinister and, ultimately, unachievable. It really stands for the expectation that we need to behave in a particular way regardless of whether it matches who we internally are. Behavior is considered "good" when it conforms to an outer standard, either that of another person or of society as a whole.

In their own way, boys also have a standard of conformity. We all do. Culture forces its children to conform and thereby raises us to be inauthentic. Girls just have it inordinately harder because we are trained to only receive validation for being good in order to perpetuate the power of the patriarchy. "Good" for women means subservient, lesser-than, not equal. Boys? They can be good or bad. In fact, sometimes the "badder" they are, the more validation they receive. They can even become the president of the United States.

To deconstruct this problem, we must get rid of the idea that there is a standard of goodness, banishing it completely. Minus such a standard, everything changes as we recognize that the idea of a standard of goodness is toxic. The notion that we are good enough *only* if x, y, and z are met is dysfunctional and must be abandoned. When we believe such a lie, we try to fit the standard in order to feel valuable. We weigh ourselves constantly on an unremitting scale of bogus numbers and comparisons.

By building her esteem around how she is seen in relationships, the good girl buys into the belief that unless she puts the others in her life before herself, she isn't caring or nurturing enough. If she doesn't appease others, she is thought of as selfish and cruel. If she happens to be bossy and demanding, she is branded a "bitch."

Of course, not everyone follows society's mandates blindly. Many give up around adolescence, either withdrawing in apathetic underperformance or striking back in rebellion. Do you remember what you did as a young woman? Did you blindly comply and morph into the epitome of "the good girl"? Or did you find yourself entering a period of listlessness and apathy? On the other hand, perhaps you became an all-out rebel?

Regardless of how it outwardly manifested in the teens and beyond, the important realization is that there is an archetype we have been conditioned to follow. Whether we rebel against it or comply with it isn't as crucial as the awareness of what we are fighting against or fleeing from in the first place.

No matter what your unique manifestation as an adolescent or adult, you can be sure that your first indoctrination as a little child resulted in the triple need for *approval, validation,* and *praise.* This is how the good girl grows up, forgetting she exists as an individual in her own right. She is trained to exist *only in context.*

Trapped in Resentment

If we are women, we share a common backstory. It doesn't matter that I am brown and you are white, or if I swaddle curves and you are lean muscle. If we are women, we share a common core. Because of this, in some fashion or another, each one of us has been afflicted by the patriarchy. This is just the by-product of being female in the modern era.

Since my own story illustrates how brainwashing works, subtly burying my essence six feet under, let me share some key aspects of the society in which I grew up with you. Whatever your own background, you will quickly realize how much we have in common.

The Black Lives Matter movement is in the news as I write. I grew up in a culture that openly and unabashedly idolized white skin. The most popular face cream was called *Fair and Lovely.* It's still a bestseller even as you read this. Brown-skinned Indian girls are taught early that their skin color is not the ideal standard. Nor is the texture of their hair, the span of their hips, or the length of their legs. Everything they find themselves to be is just not good enough. Enter facial bleaching, liquid dieting, and hair straightening.

I was given way too much attention because of my lighter skin and eyes in a country that idealizes such traits. Despite being lighter than my peers, I still didn't feel light enough and thus grew up with a liberal dose of self-loathing, forever comparing myself to the white standard of beauty I saw plastered on magazine covers and the silver screen.

The external validation my looks received as a child left me thoroughly confused. I was given extreme attention, especially by older men, while I also received scorn and disdain, mostly from older women, all before I was ten years of age. I remember thinking, "How can I make myself ugly or degrade myself enough so no one is upset with me for all the attention I receive?"

My best friend at the time later told me how it was for her to be by my side in those early days. "Walking with you on the road was the worst experience for me," she said. "You would get all this attention. People would stop to comment on your eyes or pinch your cheeks, whereas no one even glanced at me. It was like I was invisible." I remember feeling wretched when she told me this. I felt the need to apologize, to reduce myself to something lower in her eyes so she would feel better.

How must it have been for my friend to feel as if she wasn't the pretty one simply because she had dark eyes and darker skin? How messed up is a culture in which young girls grow up feeling lesser than another because they don't match an idealized standard of beauty?

The point is that many girls are plagued by this "whitified" standard of beauty. The reason is that women are incessantly judged—either exalted or denigrated—for our looks, which are out of our control. Any time our sense of worth is tied to something external, we are basically screwed. We feel good when we're validated and crappy when we aren't.

We can't help but resent other women who have what we think we need in order to feel worthy. This resentment from females in my life wasn't new to me. My young ears heard innumerable snide comments from women about my looks. One of our neighbors, who I fondly called "auntie," often warned me, "Don't think your looks will last. You are just young right now." She may have meant this compassionately, but I only heard her scorn and disgust. Little did she realize that I began to loathe my looks and simply wished I was like everyone else.

By the time I turned eleven, I had found a way to deal with the problem. I would become fat. As ironic as this sounds, this is a common approach for women who are trying to shrink themselves to a point of invisibility. This was my strategy and it worked. Finally, I was being left alone. Although men still seemed to be attracted, I stopped being resented by women. Above all, I wanted people to stop being mean to me. I wanted them to like me.

By the age of thirteen, I was fully indoctrinated into the hall of shame and subservience. I learned from the women around me that I was never to fully shine or take up too much space. The funny thing is, I didn't learn this from the men in my life so much as from the women. It was their scorn and disdain that taught me that it's far more advantageous to be a wallflower than to stand out. It was better to follow the road most traveled—maybe finish college and work a few years but, definitely and swiftly, get married, settle down, and have babies.

The road ended there, as if wifehood and motherhood were a woman's ultimate destination. To veer from this path felt threatening. Why would any woman commit social suicide? It was far easier to just swallow the pills meted out at every baby shower and follow the way of *That Woman*.

It's important that we observe our inner script around these standards and examine the toxic fallout they create. Only when we notice the emotional ravages meted out by a culture designed to suppress our natural ways do we start uncovering our authentic self. The first steps on this path involve awakening to the many ways culture has us in the grips of an unrelenting somnolence.

Becoming *That Woman*

If you really think about it, you will realize how riddled with angst women are, whatever their background or culture. The thousand things we do to our hair to give it luster and volume, the lengths we go to shape and color our nails with hues and glitter, the unspeakable amount of money we spend on makeup, and the number of YouTube tutorials we watch on how to trick the shape of our face all speak to our monumental inner disconnect.

We cover our inner void in many ways: endless diets, push-up bras, Botox treatments, fake lashes. Add to this the slimming undergarments we wear to create a body we don't naturally have, the thongs we don to accentuate the shape of our buttocks, the clothes we incessantly agonize over, or the insanely uncomfortable shoes that we adorn our feet with. All told, the amount of energy we expend anxiously "fixing" our external appearance is staggering. Of course, many of us rebel against this and go the other way in an effort to thwart "the standard." When we do, we often throw the baby out with the bath water, ignoring self-care altogether.

The inner void a woman feels, regardless of her particular background, emanates from the fact that her essence was undermined from the very start. In one way or another, her spirit was crushed. We have been brainwashed with the idea that our existence can only be fulfilled by fitting an impossible standard of goodness and beauty, which, for many of us, happens to be perfection. Perfection, of course, is relative. It basically means feeling *the pressure to be more of what you aren't.*

The standard of goodness manifests in more ways than our looks. There are the ways we stifle our voice and silence ourselves during a conflict. We are terrified of being independent in our thinking and style, so we dumb ourselves down. There are also the ways in which we cannot say no because we are afraid of retribution. These all undermine the vast treasure trove of inner power we possess but never access.

These ways of being are not explicitly taught. They don't have to be at all. As I said earlier, they just come down the pike, through the ether, passed on via the umbilical cord of the mother to the daughter. We absorb the attitudes around us through osmosis.

Because this generalization crosses all cultures, we think it is the natural way for a woman to be—the way of *That Woman*.

What I intend to show you is that all of this, *all of it*, isn't natural but purely cultural. I want to show you how we are being grossly manipulated into doing much of what we do by an unconscious culture. Then I want to illustrate how we don't have to buy into it *at all*.

I know what you are thinking, "Great pithy maxims, but hardly a reality." My own addiction to the idea of *That Woman* enslaved me for the first forty-two years of my life. It bound my throat closed so tightly that the only sound I made was a falsetto whisper. It suffocated my ribs in its tight corset. It stilettoed itself in high heels under my fragile ankles. It turned my audacious statements into whimpering questions of doubt and my truths into bald-faced lies. It covered the skin on my face, replacing it with masks. It punctured my serenity with unending angst as I tried to compare myself to other women.

No matter how far we live from home, who you or I become, how much we accomplish, how skinny we manage to be, or how many times we win the parenting contest, we are besieged by stereotypes endorsed by the women among whom we grew up. Those earliest archetypes are the bricks and mortar of our psyche.

This is why the early years are so pivotal. What we absorb as children forms the color of our cells and the viscosity of our blood. Our young ears and sensitive minds listen carefully to how our mothers claim their authority or fail to do so, and how our fathers use or abuse their power. The earliest archetypes we are surrounded with become our own. They become the foundation upon which we stand.

The only way to outgrow these archetypes is to shatter them. The only way to shatter them is to eviscerate every false identity they have created within us. We must die to who we have known ourselves to be so that our essence, our true self, can come alive and we can begin to live authentically.

As we know, it's no simple thing to change the old paradigm of *That Woman* into one that's completely redesigned from within. It takes gumption. We are creatures of homeostasis who, by and large, covet complacency over adventure and constancy over chaos. It's only when we are infused with a spirit of the wild and are ready to disrupt our lives that we are able to transform the old into something profoundly different.

I am talking about a true spiritual renaissance, the kind that takes intense inner valor and is the work of spiritual warriors. The kind of transformation I am referring to requires *a radical awakening.*

3

Do We Dare to Own Our Part?

If the sheath weren't occupied by the sword, it would lie vacant
If the quiver didn't hide the arrows, it would lie bare
If the shell didn't shroud the oyster, it would lie hollow
Each needs the other for value and purpose
Neither is complete without the other.

While women seem fated to follow cultural mandates, the power to rewrite our destiny lies within us. This is where our radical awakening plays a role. The more we acknowledge our painful emotional past, our slumber, and our psychological addictions, the more equipped we are to transcend them. Facing our inner demons is the only way to slay them. Only when we examine them one by one can we really take our power back.

This book could be a trite compilation of pithy ideas tailored to motivate women to be their best selves or to appease angry women. It could be a collection of inspirations on how we should take our power back. Books of this sort have been written by many women. I am not interested in motivating people. What I am focused on is a woman's awakening, which is something far different. Until we deconstruct how we got where we are, motivational words will not stick. They are just Band-aids, not a cure. To wake up, we need to go beyond the desire to be happy, motivated, or positive. These are wonderful qualities, but unless we are willing to do the inner work, we will simply cycle back and forth between highs and lows. It is only through our radical inner healing that we will fully enter a new birth.

The first step in this *inner work* is to go inward, just as the term implies. Our instinct is to look outward. To engage in inner work means to extricate ourselves from the external. A large part of our spiritual awakening involves a painful and arduous process of truth and reconciliation. In fact, the truth and reconciliation process postapartheid in South Africa and after the Nazi era in Germany involved exactly this—a painful retelling of the stories of abuse and pain, oftentimes in front of the perpetrators. This process honored the healing that occurs when we allow space for our wounds to be witnessed, retold, recorded, and repaired. It begins with a brutal confrontation of our suffering. Without this, there is no getting to joy. True healing always involves a full-on acknowledgment of our pain.

Skipping this process is to engage in *spiritual bypassing.* This term implies the avoidance of painful emotions in order to give ourselves and others the appearance of spiritual superiority. The truth is that we cannot "out spiritualize" ourselves by forcing ourselves to feel good. This is actually the opposite of the goal of spiritual warriorship.

Feeling exposed and vulnerable, countless female clients feel ashamed to tell me about their inner worlds. They believe they are the only ones going through these experiences. If I could give you a dollar for every story that is almost identical to the ones here in the book, you would be extremely wealthy. That's how common and universal our internal experience is. It's the way of our sisterhood. Once we realize our bond, this sorority becomes our fortitude.

If we are looking to blame others for our reality as women, we don't have to look too far. We can easily blame men and the patriarchy. It's easy to fall into a pattern of man-bashing. But to do so is misguided. When we do this, we alienate our brothers. Yes, men are a part, parcel, and leaders of the patriarchy—even its creators—but this doesn't mean they aren't also at its mercy. Because patriarchal systems have fomented over eons of time, a boy growing up today is going to feel as mired by culture's patriarchal tentacles as does a girl. Does he enjoy more privileges than she? Certainly. But my point remains—men, not just women, are subjugated by the patriarchy in their own way.

I would be remiss if I did not state that I know countless men who feel as if they have to live behind a facade. They have to hide their tears, their fears, and their sexuality. They have to don the role of provider and protector despite their authentic desires. They wear the masks of aggression or stoicism even when they might not want to. While I will continue to focus on the female experience, I don't want us to forget that we are not the only ones enslaved to the patriarchy. Such is the way of a toxic system—everyone suffers. When one is inauthentic, everyone loses. Similarly, when one breaks free, we learn that everyone has the capacity to do so.

The awakened woman doesn't understand her plight in order to bemoan it or to feel victimized by it. She takes into consideration all elements of her situation. In fact, at times, she honors how she is a beneficiary of the patriarchy. For example, she is not expected to do the menial heavy-duty manual jobs that men are expected to do. Women and children are always told to escape a dangerous situation first. Not to mention how men are more expected to fight in wars than we are. In these ways, women enjoy certain privileges that men don't, and these need to be considered as well.

Protesting against culture or the patriarchy may feel like a relief on one level but doing so also ensnares us. Whenever our cure is bound to another, even if it's justified, we stay enslaved to them. True freedom has nothing to do with the other. When we realize this, we begin to march on our path alone. This may feel impossible at first, but it isn't. It just requires a maverick inner awakening.

The wise know well that there is never solely one side to an issue. Both men and women create, maintain, and perpetuate the failures of the other. We women are cocreators of the system that subjugates us as much as we are its pawns. Part of our being in this mess is because we contribute to its continuance.

For us women to achieve a state of inner freedom, we need to acknowledge our part in the patriarchy. Unless we do, we will continue to focus on only one side of the issue, which is what *men* have done to us. While it is true that men have indeed done much against women, such as violating our freedoms, abusing our bodies, and objectifying us, it hasn't been entirely without our coparticipation. Yes, we need to educate our fathers, brothers, and sons about what their ancestral legacy holds in terms of being male. But this is not where our true and ultimate transformation lies. It begins with the question, What have we done to *ourselves*? How have we internalized the external perpetration and created an inner abuser?

Gandhi taught the Indians that the British Empire didn't hold the key to their freedom. Instead of railing against the empire to give up their two-hundred-year rule, he focused on empowering Indians. Rather than fighting the enemy, he roused the dormant inner power of the perceived "victims" by challenging the Indian people to become their own leaders. He advocated self-governance and self-reliance. Instead of relying on English textile mills, Indians began to weave their own cotton threads for their clothes, learned to produce their own salt, and refused to use foreign-made goods. He taught the Indians to honor the work of their own hands and to take pride in their accomplishments. This rendered the British occupation irrelevant.

This is what a conscious uprising looks like. It makes the oppressors irrelevant. It asks the oppressed to look at the ways *they* have participated in the perpetuation of their own subjugation by asking, How can I end the ways I am supporting my own degradation? How can I look within myself for solutions to my disempowerment?

Many women stay ad nauseam in dysfunctional relationships because they keep waiting for the other person to change. Their happiness swings like a pendulum, forever dependent on the other. This other could be anyone or anything—their parent, spouse, child, their weight, their bank balance, or beauty.

This is why couples are often miserable in their marriages for decades, or why people stay addicted to substances. It's because somewhere deep down they haven't taken full responsibility for their own dysfunctional participation in the dynamic. They have given their power to the other and in some magical fashion keep waiting for Prince Charming—or a Princess Charming, if they are attracted to the same gender—to arrive. Only when they realize he or she isn't coming do they awaken to their own inner liberator.

How many people do you know whose lives are like a yo-yo? They go back and forth constantly, forever equivocating. I could confidently say that almost all my clients come to me in a yo-yo state. And the prime reason they stay this way? They are fully convinced that the "other" is the problem.

The yo-yo isn't between ourselves and the other. We think the yo-yo is between our love and hate for the other, or our desperate need and desperate loathing for the other. It isn't. The yo-yo is between our love and hate for our own missing parts. We are waiting for ourselves. Only after much work on ourselves does the yo-yo become still. When we realize that both the problem and the solution lie in ourselves, the process of change begins. This is the missing piece, the key ingredient. Without this, even if the other person changes, we render ourselves beholden to their change.

When we see ourselves as our own enslaver, we create a path toward liberation. Full emancipation first begins in our own minds, independent of the other. When we release all external tethers, we unbridle our inner power and free ourselves to be unapologetically autonomous.

We women need to rewrite our narrative. We need to examine our entire conditioning so that we can undo the damage of centuries of patriarchal toxicity. It is in the full and bold acknowledgment of sexism that women need to rise up to ask, How do *we* perpetuate the paradigm?

The lion of patriarchy is fed on a diet of female servility. While we can bemoan the lion's predation, the wise understand that this approach is futile. True wisdom arises when we ask how this servility is perpetuated by the woman who allows herself to be internally

vanquished. Turning the focus away from how the patriarchy creates servility to how the servile create their own bondage is the only
way to break free.

How can someone subjugate us on the *outside* if we don't allow it
somewhere on the *inside?* Dominance by men involves submission
by women. Let me be clear, I didn't say that we *ask* for the submission nor even *condone* it. I said, we are *involved* in the forces that
keep these dynamics strong. As a woman, and a petite woman at
that, I am well aware of just how a man can overwhelm me with his
size without a care and that no matter how mentally strong I am,
there is really nothing I can do about it. Yet, I also know that solely
focusing on the demise of abusive male dominance is foolish, as I
will be waiting forever. The truth is this: it is only when we women
end our silence, join together as one, and raise ourselves into the
powerhouses we truly are that we will end our part in this dynamic
and transcend the clutches of the toxic patriarchy we live in. The
kind of power I am referring to rises from deep within us—from
our blood, sweat, and tears. It is from the underbelly of our deepest
suffering that we will free ourselves from our chains, one link at a
time.

Many protest when I talk about cocreation. To understand cocreation means to audaciously own our part in a dynamic, whether
by commission or omission. What I am inviting all women to do
is own their part in the dynamic so that the wheels of change can
begin to turn toward our regency.

If you are reading this and feel resistance, I invite you to notice
it and journal about what is coming up for you. Then I ask you to
keep on reading. My vision will become clearer as the pages turn. I
am not anti-woman, and neither am I anti-man. The ground I stand
on is neutral, knowing that it is only when both sexes are held in
equal esteem, with compassion and understanding on both sides,
that a lasting harmony can arise.

When my friend Sarah called me one day to say she was starting therapy, I was thrilled. *Finally,* I thought to myself. She had
suffered in an unhappy marriage for years. She then said, "I need

my therapist to teach me how to deal with my narcissistic husband. I need tools on how to talk to him!" While it was true she needed tools, I reminded her, "At the end of the day this has nothing to do with him. This is all about you—how you attracted him into your life and how you kept him engaged in a cycle of dysfunction. If you focus on him, you will lose. You need to focus on your inner void, since this is what keeps this dynamic alive."

Sarah felt as if she had been slapped in the face. Her initial anger dissipated and she shook her head slowly as it dawned on her, "Yes, it has nothing to do with him, does it? I will keep repeating the pattern and attract another narcissist into my life unless I understand *my* patterns."

In virtually every struggle my clients share with me, I inevitably hear blame. In a weird way, we derive comfort from someone else being the one who created our situation. Yet the more we blame another, the more we abdicate our power. We reduce our own power when we believe ourselves so fragile as to be broken by another. No one can break us unless we bequeath them this privilege.

Power in Our Sisterhood

Women need other women. We desperately need each other. We need our sisters to revel in our accomplishments and empathize with our struggles. We need our sisters to embrace us when our homes are untidy because we are too exhausted to clean them, and to understand us when we show up for our kids' parent-teacher meetings late or disheveled or when we forget to show up at all. We need our sisters to love us when we show up at a party in wrinkled clothes because we were up all night taking care of a sick child. We need them to be our salve, our balm, and our safe zones. Sadly, this is not always the case. Most often women feel the most judged by other women. Until this reality changes, the patriarchy will reign powerful and strong.

Each time we don't applaud a woman's efforts for simply showing up exactly as she does, we genuflect before the patriarchy. Each time we try to out-compete our sisters, we give men the message that their attention on us is our lifeblood. Instead of joining together with our naturally aging faces and saggy bottoms, we compete with one another and make our sisters feel bad about themselves. Our strength as a collective won't come from injecting more Botox so we look better than other women. Our strength will come from our sisters' embrace. This is the true calling of all feminist movements—to get women to see their strength as a collective.

Each time we knock another woman down, we are giving our power over to men—a power that they didn't ask for but will certainly indirectly benefit from. Most men I meet tell me how confused they are by how jealous and petty women can be toward one another. Remaining in competition with our sisters actually injects steroids into the patriarchy. By feeling threatened by each other we eat away at our inner vitality, which then causes us to fall prey to the patriarchy even more. The cycle of subjugation to male dominance continues on without our conscious awareness.

As we begin to wake up, our views of other women change. They no longer pose a threat or competition but instead grow into our much-needed allies. We move away from being one another's harshest critics to one another's greatest support. The feminist and other movements challenge us to become autonomous and to reduce our dependency on men. This is vital, yes, but the true pathway doesn't involve going against men—not at all. The true pathway is carved when we sisters join together as one and then widen our embrace to include the men.

Belonging to a sisterhood means to dare to be ourselves just as we are. It means to dare to speak our truth even when we fear ostracism. We dare ourselves to be transparent, allowing our authenticity to set us free. If our lives are imperfect, we embrace it. We don't fake it just for the sake of appearing perfect. We allow ourselves to be as natural as possible, as accepting and as nonjudgmental as we can be. We teach one another what it means to be self-celebratory by honoring our differences instead of trying to be the same. As we unite, we enter our inner empowerment to a greater degree, and this self-honor creates a powerful ripple effect in helping to equalize the playing field.

Our power isn't against any man. True power is never against anyone. If it was, it wouldn't be power; it would be weakness. True power is always over the self, whereas pseudopower is over the other. When we rise in true power, we will not only take care of ourselves, but also our brothers and our children. It all starts by us ending our rivalry and competition and instead upholding, mobilizing, and elevating one another.

~

4

Unmasking the Lies
We Have Been Told

The deer doesn't bemoan not being the jaguar
Nor does the daisy wilt near the rose
The lioness doesn't shrink low before the lion
Nor does the peacock dim its plume before the hawk
Each embraces its right to worth without question or doubt.

In my mind's eye, I can still be transported to my grandmother's bedroom watching her adroitly tie her sari, with its complex design, then observing her tie her long hair into a swift knot.

My grandmother never looked at herself in the mirror. One day I asked her why. She replied, "I am a widow now. This is why I only wear white saris. My youth and beauty are fading. There is no need for me to look at myself and do up my face. Those days are over. If my husband was here, it would be another thing."

I remembered not knowing whether to marvel at her sacrifice or protest. Part of me knew that this couldn't be right. Yet there she was, content with her belief that this was her fate. My deeply ingrained respect for my elders kept my lips sealed and my head nodding in agreement. Another part of me silently cried for her.

My grandmother believed in what she was doing. She believed she was right in abandoning her self-interest and living as a vestige of her former self. She believed she was no longer worthy of sexual enjoyment. She believed that this abnegation was the stairway to heaven. This was not only a sacred duty but a spiritual calling, one she fully wanted to fulfill for her own sense of identity. She had so associated her identity with sacrifice, she couldn't separate the two.

I ask myself, Was she any different from most women? Don't most of us tie our worth and well-being to how much we live for another, so much so that if we aren't giving of ourselves, we feel guilty, as if we need to defend ourselves?

While it is natural for women to bear the onus of family life because we are biologically more primed to nurture, this is the source of much conflict in the modern era, especially if a mother has desires to extend herself beyond her nurturing role. Because we are no longer living in nomadic tribal communities in the jungle, this leads to doubt, guilt, and resentment that her male counterparts are able to simply saunter past. She bears the weight of this dilemma, and often must choose either to follow her own purpose or be a wife and mother. Doing both comes at the high price of exhaustion and inner strife. As it attacks her ideas of what it means to be "a perfect woman," following her autonomous purpose feels sacrilegious and blasphemous. The price is a wretched one indeed.

The Pill That Kills

If we were to dissect a woman's brain and examine the messages ingrained therein, we would be shocked at not only how similar our beliefs are but also how many nuances we have embraced concerning how to be a woman. It's hard for us to accept that we have been utterly brainwashed. It's as if our minds have been possessed.

The main ingredient of the pill we swallow as women is that of unworthiness. This pill slowly but surely eviscerates our sense of self. While every human probably suffers from some sense of unworthiness, women have swallowed bucketfuls. The deadly part of this is that our unworthiness is heavily disguised, so much so that we often mistake it for virtuosity. This is how clever culture is. It cloaks its messages of unworthiness as virtue. For women, it's always connected to how self-sacrificing we are and how well we keep others happy. If we are unable to keep them happy, we feel like failures and therefore are unworthy.

No one needed to tell me what was expected of me as a woman. I knew by the age of five. I knew I was expected to be a good cook, to keep my house immaculate, and to raise my children well. As I grew older, the list of expectations grew as long as the Nile. Skinny, beautiful, fashionable, compassionate, and generous were added. Then there were bonus items such as having good skin, a good figure, and beautiful, long, and lustrous hair. Of course, these mandates are more from a Westernized, industrialized culture, and perhaps a woman in the rice paddies of Thailand may not experience the same indoctrination. However, she will most likely be subject to a power differential in her male–female relationships that borders on toxic and be asked to play roles that aren't authentic to her.

The mandate to be inauthentic begins at birth. Our mothers tuck these cultural dictates around the cozy sheets of our cribs and place them in the batteries of the mobiles that hang over our heads. We never question them—we never thought we had to. We are so naive as young children that we blindly trust our elders. If they tell us to pray to a certain God and we watch them do so, we are going to do this as well. If they tell us that people are not to be trusted, then we are going to follow their belief. If they tell us that brown skin is inferior and such people should leave our country, we are not only going to just believe them and think in the same vein, we are going to actually believe we are being good children by attacking brown people. If we are taught that same-sex relationships are wrong, then we become homophobic. We marry society's vision of how to be. Any diversion from it causes inner turmoil.

As children, we immediately pick up on when our parents give us a look of pride or disgust. We pick up their verbal and nonverbal cues intuitively. Reading them is like reading a map in the desert. It's our survival guide. The more sensitive we are as children, the more cues we pick up and the more we distort and contort ourselves to become the model child they desire. When we receive their validation and love, we feel reinforced and do more of what pleases them. When we are young, we will do almost anything to receive approval.

When children are squelched in this way, their suppressed feelings are buried for the moment, but these feelings don't disappear. They simply show up in their body image, self-image, grades, eating behavior, or other aspects of self-care. When we are asked to lie to ourselves, something dies within us.

Because I had grown up in a culture that plagued girls with these messages, I swore I wouldn't raise my daughter with any of them. While I'm sure a few things trickled through—how could they not?—for the large part, I consciously kept most of the robotically conditioned things out of her mind's eye. I tried as best I could to keep her untouched by cultural indoctrination.

In every woman's infrastructure lie endless familial and cultural prescriptions. The sights and smells of our culture—the good, bad, and ugly—don't voluntarily leave us. They fill our minds with images and ideations that affix themselves to our identity. Only when we separate who we are authentically from who we have been told we are, do we begin to live a life of honesty, courage, and truth.

The Noose of Expectations

When my client Megan found out she was unable to become pregnant, she fell apart. She entered a dark and deep depression. Until this moment of reckoning, it had been inconceivable to her that she would not fulfill her yearning to be a mother. What ensued was a breakdown. It was as if someone had told her she had only a few days to live.

When she finally came to see me, she appeared haggard. She simply couldn't imagine a life other than the one she had envisioned for herself. When I suggested surrogacy, adoption, or in vitro, she was unable to assimilate these options. For her, the fact she wasn't biologically endowed to become a mother made her feel she was lesser-than. Her psyche was entrenched in the idea that the only legitimate way to be a mother was if she was to birth her own children without artificial aids. It took us months to unravel this assumed identity, allowing her to discover she was worth more than just her capacity to bear children. She eventually surrendered to adopting a baby girl and grew to love her as her own.

The reason Megan's story stays with me is that she is not unlike thousands of us. Somewhere deep in our unconscious we have a vision of how we are supposed to be and the roles we are to fulfill. When this version of ourselves doesn't pan out, we go through a pivotal identity shock. We die to ourselves. We feel as if we are no one and that our life has no meaning. Who are we without the image we embraced of ourselves?

Megan's story echoes in the heads of women across the globe right now. It echoes within you to some degree or the other, begging the question, Who am I without my roles? Who am I without my identity as a wife, partner, sister, mother, daughter, friend?

Just the other day I was counseling a mother who was experiencing angst over her daughter's anxiety issues. "She feels as if she's a failure," Kate bemoaned. "She isn't the best student or the best athlete. She isn't the skinniest or the most popular. She constantly beats herself up. She feels worthless."

Kate isn't the only mother grieving over her daughter's loss of self-worth. Thanks to social media, millions of us watch our children, girls especially, become enslaved to egregious ideas of what it means to be a woman. Where before our children learned from our individual unconsciousness or that of close relatives, now they are absorbing messages from the unconsciousness of millions of other girls and women who are lost and confused. Where before the problem was focused within one's family, now the causes and effects are global. Before, grandma may have commented on the few extra pounds she put on since Easter, but now the entire world can voice their opinions of her. The result? Our young girls are more trapped than ever.

All of this shifting and morphing happens unconsciously. No one really needs to say a word. Just talk to any teenager to know that this is the way it is.

Alison, my sixteen-year-old client, felt strongly that her mother would disapprove of her if she knew she had a boyfriend. "It's as if she thinks I'm made of wood. She thinks I don't know any boys or that I shouldn't have normal feelings toward boys. Just because she didn't like boys when she was my age, she thinks I should be the same. It's so frustrating because I'm not allowed to go out with my friends, who happen to be boys, because she thinks it's inappropriate."

When I probed about how she handles the situation, she replied, "I pretend. I totally fake it. I make up lies as I go. My whole life is now a facade. When I meet Jake, I just tell my mother that I'm at Rebecca's, which means that Rebecca needs to lie as well. I have no choice. I have this whole other life that my mother doesn't know about."

From our parents and culture, we learn to lie. This is ubiquitous human behavior. There isn't a single human who hasn't learned to lie by an early age. Some become connoisseurs of mass deception, while some others resort to a few lies once in a while. Most of us grow up with the realization that telling the truth is simply too dangerous a proposition, occasioning threats of ostracism, expulsion, rejection, and abandonment. As children, we learn that telling the truth is simply not as noble as it's made out to be. The price we pay when we tell the truth is often disastrously high. As we grow up and are indoctrinated by more and more rules, our ability to tell the truth subsides even more.

The truth about lying is that it chips away at our core and tears us at the soul level. It makes us live a double or triple life that squelches our authentic self, not only with those we lie to directly but also in other areas of our life. Each time our truth gets buried, we engage in an act of betrayal toward ourselves. With every ensuing burial comes a greater and greater distrust and disconnection from ourselves. Our authentic self realizes that it doesn't have a comrade in us. We don't have our own back. We then ex-perience a great darkness of the soul, which in modern verbiage is labeled *depression*. At the soul level, depression is a deep self-abandonment.

Think about how it must feel to "live in the closet" for one's entire life. Our LGBTQ+ sisters and brothers know only too well. What fear they must face in "coming out," what dread of ostracism and invalidation! For years they have had to suppress their true self-expression, causing them to live in constant terror in terms of their safety and well-being.

Maia, my daughter, was around twelve years old when we, her parents, were in a "teaching moment" with her. We were trying to explain to her how we thought something she had done was wrong. She listened intently. I thought our message was sinking in and re-member feeling righteous. After we were done, she looked at us with a deadpan expression and said, "You know what, guys. I just realized I don't have to agree with you both. In fact, your opinion is irrelevant." After which she left the room. Our mouths were agape.

"What was that about?" my then-husband blurted out. He was mad. "Let me call her back and tell her she cannot talk to us like that!" He thought she had been utterly disrespectful. I was about to go with his plan, but then I stopped myself. I went into my big mind and realized that what she had said was actually a conscious parenting goal, involving a jewel of an insight we want every child to have. The only problem was it was hard to hear from a mere twelve-year-old. The truth is, our opinions *should* become increas-ingly irrelevant to our kids as they grow up and get to know their own minds and hearts. We should fade in their consciousness as central figures. They shouldn't have to take care of our feelings as they march forward in their lives, rising as the central protago-nists in their own journeys, mighty and powerful.

This is a fact most parents have a hard time swallowing. We didn't end up reprimanding Maia because when we distilled her comment, she had not said anything wrong—it just felt wrong to our egos. She had simply spoken her truth.

Loyalty to Traditions

Children are born into legacies, traditions, and institutionalized ways of being. If the ancestors did things in a particular way, then this is expected of the children. In the name of tradition, they are robbed of their right to discover their authentic voice and manifest their unique destinies.

Blind obeisance to tradition leads to our first and primal internal divorce from our authentic selves. From this first betrayal, springs all other forms of betrayal. Married to traditions, we believe we are committing a crime, or worse still a sin, if we go against them. Yet it is only when we see how insidious traditions can be that we dare to detach from them. Traditions are, in their own way, pressure from dead people. Bequeathed to us as if they are law, we believe we are bad for breaking them. In truth, they are just ways of being that keep us tethered to conformity and predictability. They provide us with a sense of control in an uncontrollable universe.

People who come from traditional families balk at this idea. I don't blame them. The attachment to their ways of being is so strong that what I say naturally evokes resistance, if not indignation. If you feel you are rubbing up against my message in a way that causes friction, I advise you to pause. Your resistance isn't arising because you are hearing alien ideas that are untrue or unwise. It's arising because you maybe are holding tightly on to your established ways. The tighter your hold, the greater your resistance will be to what I'm sharing with you. I advise you to be compassionate with yourself as you witness your resistance and try to ask yourself, Why am I so afraid of letting go?

Traditions, while beautiful in maintaining legacies of culture, also have the capacity to block our conscious awareness. When we grow up in an environment heavy with tradition—be it in the form of educational legacies or religious roots or cultural practices—our psyche identifies with these traditions. The more heavily traditions are placed on our young shoulders, the more we fuse our identity with them—so much so that we are soon incapable of knowing who we are outside of these traditions.

We like to think of ourselves as having free will, but our free will is akin to eating at a buffet at which our choices are limited to the skills and preferences of the owner of the restaurant and the chef. We make choices within the choices already made by others. For a long time, we don't even make those choices, but blindly swallow the crumbs our parents and culture set down for us. Our clothes, the God we worship, our profession, and perhaps even our spouse are predestined for us by the families we are born into. Owning up to the degree to which our choices have been stolen from us is key to our awakening.

We think we choose marriage, our careers, our religion. We don't. None of these choices is purely ours. Only when we understand how our lives are fueled by traditions from the past can we hope to free ourselves from the moorings of robotic conformity.

I long ago realized that many traditions, particularly Indian ones, while beautiful and certainly worthy of keeping according to a person's free choice, were filled with subscripts of subjugation, servility, and patriarchy. The problem is not in the traditions per se but in how they are presented to us as the Holy Grail. The fact that these traditions are tied to our sense of worth is the issue. If they were offered to us as a choice rather than as a metric of our worth, it would be another matter. The truth is that many of our traditions rob us of our innocence by dictating we follow them instead of following our own beautiful inner longings.

Leaving a tradition after having been ensconced in it for decades feels like a betrayal, even a death, which is why few leave their traditions behind. This is the same reason a gay person may endure great internal toil before "coming out of the closet." They are breaking the tradition of heterosexuality, which is the prevalent way of forming a family.

By their nature, traditions absolve themselves of creativity, spontaneity, and individual design. They are intrinsically meant to bind us to the past, obstructing a serious inquiry into how the past might or might not fit into our present or future. Instead of allowing our children and ourselves to roam in and out of traditions with ease, selecting the ones that are uniquely suited to our personality, we feel bound to honor the ones that were laid before us during childhood. When ghosts of our past live in the present, they subconsciously dictate how we live. We are handed subtle scripts about how things were and how they are "supposed to be." We presume the feeling of obligation these traditions arouse is normal.

We may claim to love a family tradition but, on closer examination, we may realize we are just habituated to it and are therefore blindly attached. The question we need to ask ourselves is, Are we keeping the tradition out of obligation or out of a genuinely conscious relationship with it? Unless we allow for this inner inquiry, we will continue to be enslaved by what came before us.

The emancipated woman is one who sees through the fallacy of being bound by tradition. She is willing to lose all of them—and I do mean *all* of them—if necessary. In due course, she may choose to keep a few, but only after she has first confronted what it means to be without them. Arriving at the barren field of possibility, where no signposts exist, she knows she has ventured home to *herself.*

5

Deconstructing Patterns

The thread of the needle creates our life design
It stitches intricate shades of confusing patterns
Crisscross, crisscross, the colors move across the tapestry
Causing us to lose sight of where it all began
Soon, we wear clothes unaware of how
the holes were stitched over.

This may be one of my most profound insights as a therapist. *We don't live a life, we live a pattern.*

I want to take you beyond the surface disruptions of your life to a deeper layer, where the patterns that drive us are always clear. The process of entering this deeper layer is like removing cobwebs from our eyes. The reason most of us don't notice our patterns is that we have been hungry for two foods, love and worth. So hungry have we been that we are in a hallucinatory stupor. Attention, acceptance, and validation are the prizes we obsess over, rabidly hunting them at all costs.

Because we believe what we are looking for can only be found on the outside, this hunt takes us from relationship to relationship and, at other times, from achievement to achievement. We feel "puppeteered" by the world and conclude that situations happen *to* us, rather than with our consensual participation. We feel like hapless bystanders, with no choice but to react to what life throws at us. We may have acted like passive reactors, yo-yoing to whatever shows up in our lives, but the truth is, we are extremely active participants in, and cocreators of, our experiences. Passivity then, is a choice—a very active one at that, disguised as a non-choice. Unless we own that our roles as passive bystanders are actually an outgrowth of an active choice, we will stay mired in them, hapless to the consequences they unleash. These patterns of passive reaction stem from how we were conditioned to seek love and worth from our parents. These patterns are a way of answering these questions:

Am I loved?
Am I seen?
Am I worthy?

Instead of discovering how to give these things to ourselves, we sought them from the external world, mainly our parents. Children everywhere are raised to seek approval and validation from their elders. Our parents are at the top of the hierarchy, of course, followed by our family's elders, and then by teachers. This sets us up to depend on them. In our desire to obtain the love and worth we feel we need from them, we readily abandon ourselves and fall in line.

No matter how many times I say this to clients, it takes many mentions for them to fully connect just how impacted their current life patterns are by their early childhood. The emotional penny takes a long time to drop. If I repeat this point throughout the book, it's for this reason: the more we hear it in different ways, the more aware we will be of our inclination to repeat our patterns.

Linda is the perfect example of someone who had spent years in therapy "doing the work" yet, for the life of her, she couldn't understand why she was riddled with anxiety at the prospect of accepting a recent promotion at work. When it was time to meet with her boss to go over details of her new responsibilities, she created the excuse she was ill. When the meeting was postponed to the following week, she created another excuse that her child was ill.

"What is wrong with me?" she asked. "This is something I have always wanted and yet, now that I am being offered it, I am terrified." Linda was stricken by a fear of failure. It took us several sessions to deconstruct the roots of her fear. Having grown up in a very religious and strict family, she learned early on that to avoid punishment, she needed to be perfect. She manifested this in all sorts of ways, including academic excellence, body fitness, marrying a successful entrepreneur, and raising her children to be high achievers. She seemed to have it all together until this moment of collapse.

Upon deconstructing her past and finding connections to the present, it was clear she thought she was going to fail at the new job. She wasn't confident. Like when she was a child, she was terrified of being punished. So enmeshed was she in her past that she was unaware of how it was affecting her present reality. Her past fears took over and she was paralyzed, like she used to be as a little girl. "When I was little, I hid in my closet, terrified of my father's anger. I would wait there till dark and only when I was sure he was asleep would I crawl out into my own bed." Linda was repeating her emotional trauma here. She was scared of being a failure and facing retribution, so she was hiding in her "closet."

I mentioned earlier that we learn through osmosis to pay attention to how our parents act toward us, contouring our behavior accordingly. Linda learned to create a persona of perfectionism to avoid punishment. However, as she grew older, this persona was paralyzing her and causing her to sabotage her own progress. As our ego comes to the fore, we do whatever it takes to get our parents to notice us. We become comedians or pleasers, angry rebels or obedient followers. We act out or act in. We passively follow or we aggressively detour. We flail and flounder, progress and regress, all in our desperate quest for love and worth. Thus begins the dance of inauthenticity. So what if we forsake our authentic self, as long as we believe we are loved? We believed that was the gold at the end of the rainbow.

Our prominent emotional experiences as a child become our template, the pattern we now unconsciously replay. These are what I call the wounded feelings left over from childhood. As a child, to feel the inner pain is too frightening. It's much easier not to feel, which is where the ego helps us by forming a hard shell around our pain, and channeling all our hurt energy into a false persona. Once we figure out our basic pattern for relating to people and events, we see it everywhere. Our patterns are most apparent when we are faced with a challenging situation, and we revert right back to the instinctual strategy we employed as a child.

In my work as a therapist, I see that we not only live a pattern, we *are* the pattern. The pattern becomes us or, another way to say it, the ego becomes us. We believe we *are* the persona we adopted in order to cope with our childhood. Rather than contouring ourselves to the newness of each moment, the moment is reinterpreted to match the old template. We no longer live in a spontaneous way, authentically responding to the moment-by-moment experiences of life. Instead, we are highly charged and reactive, swinging like a wild pendulum according to the triggers coming from the outside.

It isn't easy to see our reactivity to a difficult situation as a repetition from our past. So fused are we with our pattern that we cannot fathom how these patterns are ingrained default systems that we are injecting into the present moment. It all feels so real. Once we discover that we are repeating an emotional pattern, we can start the process of dismantling these deeply ingrained ways.

The Difference Between Authenticity and Goodness

When we notice our addiction to seeking love from the outside, we might dare to ask what it means to give *ourselves* love. What would it mean to value our own knowing so much that it occluded the opinions of others? Can we possibly honor and respect our own self that much? When we begin this serious inquiry, we might be shocked to discover how little we value ourselves. We might find ourselves saying:

No, I cannot give myself love and worth.
No, I don't trust my opinion or knowing.
No, I don't believe I am important enough to listen to.

We might notice how insignificantly we treat ourselves and how little we esteem our own inner voice. We would rather obtain significance from others before we find it within ourselves. If you sit deeply with this realization, you may realize how discarding and cruel we are to ourselves. How on earth did we learn such self-invalidation and self-loathing?

Awareness of how our inner disconnect perpetuates our disempowerment has the potential to shake us to our core. This awareness has the power to snap us out of being a victim and blaming others. Perhaps for the first time, we can see how we are the full-time stagehands in our theatrics, setting the props for our inner demise. There is no evil outer. Our significant others only play a role we cast for them in our lives. The power never lies in them, only in us.

In order to shift, we need to be aware of what is going on inside us. We need to check in with ourselves on a moment-by-moment basis, asking the following:

Am I acting out of obligation and duty, or alignment and authenticity?

Am I acting out of fear of losing another's love, or the power of self-love?

Am I acting out of scarcity of what-*if,* or abundance of the what-*is*?

Am I in lack about the future, or empowerment about the present?

Am I acting out of a desire to please the other, or a desire to please myself?

Am I acting out a past pattern, or honestly responding to the present?

Do any of our motives spring from authenticity and self-governance, or are most of them driven by an inner need emanating from the void at our center? If the latter, it's quite likely that all our motives are duty-bound, fear-based, and focused on lack. As we become aware of these inner disconnects, a realization grows that we need to pivot to a new place of inner connection. But how? What fosters a state of inner connection?

The answer always returns to inner stillness and reflection. The more we learn to sit quietly with ourselves in self-reflection, the more we become aware of what's going on within. We begin to depend on our own company and relish our own friendship. We develop a companionship with our inner being and learn to value its opinions, desires, and ideas. In essence, we begin to court our authentic self.

As we check in with ourselves, we catch ourselves in the act of self-betrayal as it's happening. When we catch ourselves about to sell ourselves short, we pivot and shift. More and more attuned to our acts of self-abnegation, we pay attention when we suppress our inner voice and, instead, begin to speak up. At first, we might not even be able to separate our voice from the din of others, but slowly we become better able to do so. It may take months or many years, but eventually, we will arrive at a new place where the needle begins to move from the outer to the inner, from self-imposed duty to authenticity, from lack to abundance, from fear to self-empowerment. The natural blossoms of these shifts is a burgeoning sense of inner love and worth. Before we know it, we begin to hold ourselves in the reverence we formerly accorded to others.

When this seismic shift from self-loathing to self-love completes itself, we are left with a renewed understanding of our authentic power and purpose. Finally, having reconnected with ourselves, we feel intimately connected with all life around us. This is the power of self-love and self-honor.

The Role of the Role

I pay homage to the impact of our ego throughout the book because understanding it is key to our awakening. Unless we can spot our ego in action, we will be under its control and won't ever be able to fully flourish as spiritually awakened adults.

The ego is a vital and necessary ally—I liken it to the shell of an egg, which protects the chick before and during its hatching. If the eggshell stays intact, it will eventually kill the chick it was designed to protect. The goal of spiritual growth is never to annihilate the ego or begrudge its role. The goal is only to understand it and, through this, outgrow the need for it.

When we spot our ego in action, we need to remember that it's covering up the wounds of childhood. As such, it always comes from lack. It's only when we excavate the unresolved feelings that make up this lack that we can heal what has been wounded. We begin to realize all the ways we have compensated for our pain and how these ways actually took us further and further from our truth.

Our authentic self is right within us, beneath the feelings of the hurt child. As our pain is healed by our growing awareness of who we really are, our truth emerges bright and clear. The path of healing involves recognizing the ego's facades in our patterns and learning to pause when we see them. The pause allows us to ask the questions that allow us to go deeper. We need to ask, What is the ego protecting? How can I help soothe my childhood issues so I don't need to employ a false persona?

Just by pausing and turning the spotlight on the ego's ways, we automatically channel our energies away from them. The ego begins to weaken. Our focus goes where it's needed. Our childhood gets a chance to voice its fears. Unlike what happened in childhood, this time it's *heard*. For the first time in our life, perhaps, our childhood fears are soothed.

Looking in the mirror is the hardest thing in the world. No one wants to admit that they are the cause of their own misery—no one. It's just too painful. It's much easier to go about life innocent of our own contribution. Checking in on our sneaky ego is the key. The grand chicanery of our ego's patterns is that they manifest in a different way each time, blindsiding us to the fact that *we* are the common denominator in our experiences. We get so beguiled by the ego's many facades, we take them at face value and believe them to be our real self, when in fact they are just repetitive patterns of inauthenticity.

This is why there are more failed second marriages than first marriages. People aren't aware of their patterns. Their ego makes them believe they are falling in love with an entirely different person because this person is blond instead of brunette, or this person is an accountant instead of a musician. Because the presentation is different, we believe the experience will be too. Little do we know that underneath the presentation is the same emotional consciousness that drove our last love affair.

Within months of moving on to a different relationship as a single person, or not long into a new marriage if that is our choice, the old patterns surface. Unlike the first marriage, our tolerance for bullshit the second time around is much less. Sometimes it takes several relationships for us to realize that we basically keep attracting new partners with the same old emotional patterns.

Oh, the many faces of the ego! Sometimes our patterns of behavior present as procrastination at work, a bullying boss, or an unreliable coworker. Because we haven't encountered this particular life situation before, we get swept away by the novelty of it and begin to react to these situations as if they were brand new. Over time, we begin to feel the same way we felt at our old job or life situation. We feel fatigued, restless, and bored. Or we might feel disempowered. We ask ourselves, How did I get here again? Where did this feeling come from? Why am I back to square one? It doesn't strike us that we are in what Freud called a "repetition compulsion." We compulsively repeat the same emotional experience again and again.

Self-awareness is the ego exterminator. It takes the wind out of the ego. This is why awareness is always the first step. Awareness of reality is always where we begin. We become present to our patterns. We ask ourselves:

What faces does my ego usually wear?
When is it likely to be triggered?

How does it behave when triggered?
What is the payoff it receives?
What is it trying to protect within me?

By asking the right questions, we prevent our ego from taking over and dominating our lives. Our courage to go inward and own our wholeness automatically diffuses the power of the ego, allowing it to retreat. What emerges on center stage is our more authentic self, one that is no longer afraid to be transparent, raw, and real. The days of needing to wear the ego's facades as a shield are now in the past. A new tomorrow is on the horizon.

6

Shedding Skin

There comes a moment when yesterday's girl dies
A moment when her old wounds suddenly stop bleeding
A moment when her chains suddenly melt
A moment when her quest for redemption ends
When she finally arrives at the dawn
of her spiritual renaissance.

This chapter is going to take us on several aspects of my personal journey. Although I reveal details about my unique path, I ask you to read it using your own life lens as well. Perhaps my words will allow you to see a mirror of your own trials and tribulations. When you extrapolate my experiences to your own life, they will have the most impact.

As you read, ask yourself, How does this apply to my own struggles? When have I felt similarly, and how can I use her process to elevate my own choices in life? In this deeper inquiry, this book will serve you the most. It requires an inner stillness and readiness to reflect deeply. I trust you are ready for this.

My moment of clarity was both traumatic and epiphanic. I knew with unwavering certainty that I could no longer continue in my marriage as it stood. Something needed to change—either me, my then-husband, or the whole ball of wax.

My ex-husband was the only man I had been with for twenty-two years, and I had never imagined my life without him. We had grown up together and then grown apart. Until the balance skewed toward the latter, we had been fully wedded and embedded in our relationship. For all those twenty-two years, I never looked beyond him or my marriage.

A zillion causes and effects led to the day when I woke up with the clearest understanding that my marriage needed to end. What were these causes and effects? Well, the first cause began in my own childhood conditioning, as it does with us all. These causes set up psychological structures within me that caused me to effortlessly betray myself. The effects of this internal structure created relationship patterns where I allowed my authentic power to be crushed and didn't advocate for its preservation. This paralysis riddled me with shame, which in turn caused further suppression and silencing.

My ex-husband added his own particular causes and effects from his childhood. Together we cocreated our unique marital dynamics. Our unresolved childhood wounds set up patterns where I was cast as the emotional nurturer and caregiver, trying to be the fixer, rescuer, and healer. As a result of my role reenactments, my own needs went unattended. My inner well kept drying up, creating scarcity within.

There were so many moments when I clenched my jaw in silence in order to keep the peace, so many moments where I swallowed my dignity in order to keep the family intact. When I wanted to say no, I didn't. Instead I bobbed my head in acquiescence. When I wanted to assert my will, I didn't. Instead I convinced myself that my desires were unmerited. So afraid was I to rock the boat and be seen as a troublemaker that I did everything humanly possible to keep the ship afloat. I thought to myself, If only I could be nicer, then we would be happier! If only I was skinnier, we would have better sex. If only I earned more money, we would enjoy life more. I railed against myself constantly, berating myself for not being "good enough." I was so afraid of his disapproval and withdrawal of love that I tried to become his every fantasy. So enmeshed and fused was I with his sense of well-being that I completely lost every last connection to myself.

Whenever I perceived my husband's displeasure, I ascribed

it to a lack within myself. I thought surely it must be because of something I didn't do well enough. Soon Shefali's "not good enoughness" became the story of the marriage and my inner trauma. As a result, I kept trying to be better and better. Ms. Perfecter, Ms. Gooder, Ms. Sexier. Whatever it took, I was going to do it. And then twenty-two years later it all came to a screeching halt. I hadn't noticed the gas tank had been empty for a few years. I had literally scraped the bottom of the barrel. There was literally nothing more to give. I had reached the end of my capacity.

Every couple contributes their own causes and effects. It's for each of them to dissect these dynamics for themselves. The greatest power arrives in taking ownership of our own internal causes and effects instead of blaming the other. When things don't go the way we desire, we often try our hardest to control or change the other. This is often our first line of attack. I did this for years. I kept waiting for my ex-husband to stop his patterns so I could feel relief. After many unsuccessful attempts to get him to shift, I woke up and realized the only person who needed to change was myself.

Eventually, we are hit by the epiphany that growth depends on us, not the "other." Instead of focusing on them, we need to focus on our own emotional contribution, such as, How am I reacting to the other's behavior? How are my conditioned ways of being supporting their behavior? How am I executing my choices? How am I participating in the cyclical dynamics?

In any situation, we always have three choices—to stay and accept things the way they are, to change things (either ourselves or the other), or to leave. Which do we choose? Often we cycle back and forth between these for years, unsettled and ambivalent. We realize that the power to change our lives ultimately falls on us and we are sometimes resentful of this. We begrudge the other for forcing us to make difficult choices. This is spiritually immature. No one can ever force us to choose. Our own causes and effects create the struggle. There is no one on the outside to blame. When we realize this, we end our victimhood and rise above the limitations of our past.

As I began to slowly and "inchingly" awaken, I realized that I needed to stop waiting for my ex-husband to stop his patterns and instead end my own. I needed to change what I was doing. If I thought I was giving too much, well, instead of begging him to stop taking, I needed to change myself and simply cease giving. This was the shocking and simple truth. Of course, this meant creating boundaries, something I was really terrible at. I needed to start saying no, when all these decades I had been saying yes. The seismic shocks to my marriage were profound.

As I kept growing, I began to create new causes and effects within my psychological structure and, in doing so, quite naturally left behind vestiges of the "old Shefali," and entered new iterations of myself. Different sentences began to come out of my mouth, and fresh boundaries were made. Even the food I put into my mouth changed. The way I dressed dramatically altered, the way I held my shoulders, the way I made eye contact, the way I thrust my chin when I spoke. Subtle but profound shifts were created in my external self as my internal self began to evolve. People commented that I had a new "look." Yes, it was the look of an awakened woman.

Quite naturally, the power dynamics in my marriage were shaken. The reverberations created huge cracks in the system, which led us down a crumbling path toward the great unknown. What we thought were citadels and fortresses began to topple. Soon there was rubble everywhere. It was yet to be seen whether the restoration crew could re-create a new vision for their old city.

When we change our patterns, we create dramatic upheavals in the status quo of our relationships and, quite naturally, people in the old system begin to protest. Of course they do. They want things to return to the way they used to be and, in turn, resist the changes we are making. Inevitably, there is a huge clash. At this moment, the couple has a choice about how to resolve this clash. Either the one changing stops their growth, which is typically what happens, or the one resisting stops resisting and is welcoming of the other's growth.

In my case, neither happened. Neither of us changed enough to flow with the other. The result? An emotional dam. An unresolvable situation. I think, at some level, we both knew it was futile. We had grown too emotionally distant. As tragic as this was, we realized this movement apart was inevitable.

Each step I made toward my awakened self quite naturally created deep internal strife. There was doubt and hesitation, ambivalence and fear—and, at times, downright terror. The only realization that kept me evolving was the fact that I had no other choice. Either I continued the old way and kept denying my authentic self, or I allowed this new part of me to grow and continued to forge a path of awakening.

Every aspect of my life underwent a drastic overhaul as I began to awaken—not just in my marriage but every relationship. Where before I was quiet and timid, I now dared to protest and defy. Where before I compromised and sacrificed myself, I now dared to place myself first. Where before I allowed myself to be ridden roughshod over, I now created stoic boundaries of power. And you know what two things I stopped the most? I stopped overexplaining and I stopped begging for validation.

For a long time, I had been in the habit of explaining myself in order to be seen as "good." I finally got to the place where I was okay being seen as the "bad" one. I was okay being misunderstood, even grossly misunderstood. I finally got to the place where the only person I needed validation from was myself. This was a huge inner moment of growth for me. I was okay with another being who was not okay with me. Before this would have been unthinkable. And finally, after decades, I was okay with it. It took a bloody long time for sure, but once I arrived there, oh, what a sweet victory it was! It was a welcome back to *me*.

My many profound internal reverberations had begun to change the world around me. My awakened self impacted every area of my life, including my work, and I soon began to make different decisions in my career and to take risks like I never had before. The butterfly had begun to flap her wings and was about to take flight. She could no longer be caged. Her flight to the open skies was finally unfettered and free.

The thing that happens when women awaken is that we honor ourselves. This self-honor allows us to create new standards for our lives, some that are often nonnegotiable. This creation of standards may be a daunting step, but it's vital on our path to evolution. We see life as it is and not as we fantasized as a little girl. We wake up our little girl. We shake her into her power. If disrespect is on the menu, we leave the table—no exceptions. If inauthenticity is in the air, we leave the party. Whenever our former martyr-self shows up, we gently but firmly show her the door. Big feelings are no longer to be feared, but celebrated. Life absent our thousand inner critical voices suddenly becomes clear and simple. If we wish to speak, we do. If we wish to cry, we do. There is no one to ask permission from and no one to blame. We become our own mothers, lovers, and best friends. We become our own giving tree.

Make no mistake, it took me decades to get here and I got help from many sources. I say this because I don't want to give the impression that this is a quick 1-2-3 process. Being a mother definitely made the process more challenging. The weight of this burden was, at times, almost too excruciating to bear. Mothers may feel this more heavily than their male counterparts. Since women place the responsibility of nurturing the family more firmly on their own shoulders, it causes them deep pain when they feel they are abandoning their children in some way.

I was scared to change the status quo of my marriage too much because I knew it would mean emotional distress for my daughter. At times, I wanted to stop my flight for fear it might clip her wings. Her well-being was more important than mine, without a doubt. At any moment, I was ready to halt my awakening in order to keep her comfortable. The inner conflict was high. At times it was downright torturous.

How is a mother supposed to make the difficult choice between her children's well-being and her own liberation? It's virtually impossible. The only way she can ultimately go forward is when she unequivocally believes that her path will be in the best interest for all. Only when she is fully convinced that staying, despite the immediate comfort it brings, will be more toxic than going through the fire of transformation, will she dare put another step forward.

So it was in my case. I saw my "great withering" so clearly that I knew if I stayed, I wouldn't be able to mother my daughter the way she deserved. I saw that staying was compromising my mental health to such a degree that she would be far more greatly served if I left and regained my stability. I knew I would be a way better mother and role model out of the marriage than in it.

These choices don't come easily to any of us. The path illuminates itself after years of deep self-awareness and soul searching. A true renaissance in the making, it's one that ultimately results in the evolution of all.

But what if the choice forward isn't as clear as mine was? Many women in unhappy relationships stay stuck in indecision and the status quo for years. Both the choice to stay on the ledge or to jump feel equally treacherous. They cannot find redemption in either. The question, Should I stay or should I leave? lingers over them for decades. I always tell such women that their moment to make the final choice has not yet appeared. Because fear permeates both of their choices, they can't find courage to resolve their dilemma either way. I soothe them by saying, "This is not the time. Accepting this is pivotal. When we do, we surrender to the emotional place we are in and honor its back and forth."

We now need to "sit" in this space. This "sitting" takes emotional strength and perseverance. It's not an act of defeat or passivity to "sit," but instead one of wisdom—as long as we are actively observant during the process. In fact, I talk about "sitting in it" as if it's a legitimate spiritual strategy, because for me it is. There is much to be gained from sitting with a struggle. We watch our battle with gentle kindness and allow for pros and cons to rear their heads as needed. We don't push for one side to win over the other. Both sides are here to tell their story and impart their wisdom. If we move too quickly, before one is ripe, it may be a decision made in haste, and have worse consequences later. We don't disparage ourselves or rush ourselves to a conclusion. This is an important part of the "sorting through" process. If we skip it out of an intolerance for the ambiguity it brings, we bypass important parts of our growth.

There is wisdom in doing things when the time is right. There is a lot to be said for spiritual timing. What this means is that we move forward only when there is a clear clarion call. This usually happens when our inner awareness finds its match in the outer world. Both our inner and outer reality line up. We await this alignment. Whenever the choice doesn't present itself clearly, we need to own the phrase "I am not ready just yet." We allow for the lack of clarity to be our bedfellow, trusting that through this surrender the right path will emerge when it's time to do so.

When women dare to make emboldened choices, we often fear how our partner will react. Will they respond with wrath or compassion? When it's the former, we are often faced with terror. Our physical safety may be in jeopardy. Males being stronger and more aggressive by nature have the potential to become a physical threat. It doesn't even matter if our partner is male or not. Sometimes, even when the other is a female who turns toward aggression when undergoing trauma, it can be a downright terrifying experience. Giving ourselves the space and permission to feel these fears is key to creating new pathways for ourselves. Such patterns need to be broken, first by honoring our fears and then devising ways to break free. When we allow another to oppress us in any way, fear naturally looms. Only when we see how we have handed our power over to another can we own our part and create a new narrative.

Women in physically dangerous relationships don't have the luxury of time, which is a sad, but true reality. The moment things gets physically abusive, I strongly urge my clients to leave. Here, there is no choice to be made. The choice was carved in stone after the first violation against them. It's already too late for such women. These women have a tendency to blame themselves for the danger they are in. So mired are they in their lack of self-worth, they cannot muster the self-dignity to get out of abuse. Often their children play a huge role in their fear to leave. These women, in particular, need to learn that there is a difference between fear and terror. While the former can be a natural element of any crisis, the latter is a defining signal to exit. When fear crosses into terror, even just once or twice, a woman needs to take bold action, even if it means creating an expedient exit strategy.

Our sons and daughters cannot afford to make our mistakes. They need to learn that there are ultimately no excuses for toxic behavior, no matter how "nice" the other person is most of the time. Most of all, they need to learn that they don't have to tolerate living in fear or terror of another human under any circumstance. When we embolden them with a declarative "never tolerate any form of oppression," we give them the green light to leave any abusive situation, no exceptions. No questions need be asked, and no excuses conjured. Just as they should never drive intoxicated, they should never be emotionally intoxicated in an abusive relationship. Our mandate is to help them realize the power of their choices and their right to execute them. It starts with us.

Being natural nurturers, women are reluctant to engage in choices that can cause disruptions in other people's lives. We care so much about the well-being of others that this weighs us down and clouds our decisions to take care of ourselves. In addition to being afraid of the impact my choices would have on my daughter, I was afraid of how our extended families would react. I was afraid to cast pain on both sets of our elderly parents. I considered his family my own and still do. Would they still love me? Would they be mad at me? The risk of losing connection with them was high.

Then there was my community. How would they feel? Would they judge me for not being "the conscious parent"? After all, I had written books on this, as well as one entitled *The Awakened Family*. Would the decision to leave my marriage cause my supporters to leave me as well? I drew solace from the fact that I never once described a conscious parent or an awakened family in conventional terms. If anything, I consistently underscored how authenticity was their main hallmark. I share this to bring you in on my struggles and show how I, like many of you, fell prey to enormous fear and self-doubt.

I don't want women who are reading this to fear that if they awaken, their marriages are destined to end. This is definitely not the case. Not all marriages need to dissolve like mine did just because the dynamics shifted upon the awakening of one partner. Many times, both partners are able to adapt, evolve, and grow together, entering a new marital consciousness. When this happens, it's a beautiful thing, indeed. Many partners are excited by each other's growth and seek to change themselves to stay in sync with the other. Some can do this successfully, while others cannot. There is no judgment on the ones that cannot. For the couples who can, spiritual evolution becomes a family affair. I have seen this happen many times in my practice and it's a hugely enlightening process for all.

I have talked about the role of fear in this book. If these pages have a core message, it would be about revisioning fear. I want to show you that fear was a companion on my journey to authenticity. This is natural and normal. The point of a courageous life is not to extinguish fear, per se, but to befriend and transform it. Courage is born in such a transcendence.

While living in fear of another needs to be extinguished swiftly, we need to understand that inner fear is a natural and normal part of human instinct. Many of us are afraid of fear, which is where fear wins. In my journey of awakening, I had to renegotiate my relationship to my inner fears. In doing so, I have now completely transformed how I overcome fear when it shows up. I know that each time fear raises its head, I need to allow it to be felt. Instead of running away from it or shutting it out, I need to lean into it. What is this particular fear trying to tell me? What needs healing in order for it to not feel so ominous?

I slowly began to create a new relationship with fear. Each time fear showed up, I greeted it and allowed it to constrict my chest and well up my eyes. It was beautiful because it was natural. Of course, it would often show up in unfamiliar and new ways each time. It was warning me that there were no road maps and no clear pathways. As soon as I listened and soothed my fear, it began to abate.

Do you know who was able to do that within me? My authentic self. The more I began to exercise my authentic self, the more she rose in power and strength. Soon she was holding court and managing all my chaotic inner emotions.

There is no clear-cut path to awakening. The decisions I made along the way may have worked for me, but they might be disastrous for another. The important thing to bear in mind is not to focus so much on the exact external strategies I implemented, but instead on the internal ones. Here is where universal resonance can be found. What were my fears? How did I identify them and try to overcome them? How did I negotiate my inner world? These are the keys to help women across various demographics. The external choices I made may be unique to my circumstances, but these don't stop women from learning from my internal process.

The reason I am sharing just how scary the process of awakening was for me is so that I can give other women who may be alone solace that they are not alone in their fears. It *is* a terrifying prospect to change one's life. During these times, it's imperative to seek help and counsel.

I was lucky to turn to my best friend during this process. The support I received was invaluable in helping me move forward. Together, hand in hand, we journeyed from the known into the unknown. When I forgot my inner power, my friend constantly reminded me of it. When I doubted myself and entered the blame-shame cycle, my friend held a mirror to my true self and challenged me to leave the remnants of my ego behind. When I wanted to give up and cower in fear, I was picked up and carried over to the other shore. My tears were soothed, my terrors allayed. The bright horizons of tomorrow were painted on my emotional doors. All I needed to do was open the lock and step through. These are the gifts of a wise friend.

Having a community, or even one trusted confidante, is helpful in our process. It can be hard to do it alone. In order for us to call in support, we need to first be brave enough to ask for help. We need to let it be known that we are in need and open ourselves to depending on another. This takes courage. It means we need to let go of our mantle of perfection and our superwoman status and allow ourselves to enter the humility of being needy.

Many of us struggle with this because we don't want to be a burden and because we are attached to our ideas around competency. Yet reaching out for help implies we are open to our interconnectedness and togetherness. By stepping off the pedestal of perfection, we actually sound the clarion to other women to do the same and thereby build networks of power around one another. In my journey, my closest friends were my allies and my strength. They created an invisible circle of comfort and confidence around me, without which I may not have been able to move forward with empowerment and clarity as I did.

Awakening is a beast. There is 100 percent truth to the adage that ignorance is bliss. Of course it is. It's so much easier to keep our head in the sand and follow the dictates of others. When we are silent, no one gets upset with us. Silence means we don't need to deal with the mess conflict causes, nor do we have to take painstaking actions to change our lives. Things can just stay comfortable and predictable. There is much safety in this.

For many, this bubble of ignorance will be the mainstay of their existence. But there are a few women, a few wildflowers, for whom this ignorance will become the noose around their neck causing unbearable suffering. It's for these women that I write these words.

It makes sense that the decade of their forties is the decade of metamorphosis for many women who choose to take the road less traveled. Having followed the checklist dutifully—educated, wed, and perhaps mothered—we have completely forgotten ourselves until now. But something happens when our children become teens. Watching them burst into autonomy and be bold, defiant, and confrontative wakes something within us. We are jolted into an awareness of our own passivity and docility. We watch our children be reckless, bold, and unafraid. They stop needing us as much. We begin to seriously wonder, Who am I to be now?

This is certainly what happened to me. My daughter hit thirteen and had grown into an independent and strong young woman. She no longer needed her mother in quite the same way. I went from "mommy" to "mom." Every mother knows that when this happens, it signifies the end of her unabashed power over her child's life. The child has finally figured out that mommy isn't that amazing, that smart, or that entertaining. The world is much bigger than "mommy" and needs to be explored. She is just "mom" now, a means to an end, to be beckoned only when needed for food, money, or car rides.

The year my daughter turned thirteen was the year I, too, turned my life around. She began to fly the coop and so did I. She birthed wings and so did I. The time to leave the nest had arrived. Like a pregnant woman past her due date, my own spiritual cervix dilated and nothing was the same in my world anymore.

Writing a New Narrative

We can write new narratives for ourselves, including how we look, how and if we marry, how we parent, and for whatever choices we make. This is scary at first because we find ourselves in uncharted waters, but soon we find freedom in the process. Once we realize that culture doesn't get to define us, we begin to take our power back. The validation we sought from others no longer means as much to us. We now ground ourselves in a new reality, one based on self-validation.

If there is one institution where fear rules the game, it's the institution of divorce. Culture has infused dread into the divorce process as a way of controlling people and keeping them together. The entire system is set up to foster tyranny, fear, and competition. The family court system and divorce attorneys are all primed to perpetuate this sense of dread. Divorce attorneys are trained to win battles, not tame egos or tend hearts. The smell of war permeates the entire process.

In my divorce, I knew I was facing the gargantuan task of dismantling my fears around lawyers and the court system. I knew that just as culture had created its own version of marriage, it had created its own version of divorce. Because it was a cultural artifact, I had a choice in how I interacted with it. I could either succumb to culture's way, or I could pave my own way. I saw it as my spiritual challenge to deconstruct my fears around this institution. I knew that my evolution depended on my ability to transform my relationship to fear.

I knew that unless I fought back against the stigma of divorce, I would not only fail myself, but also my daughter, and all those I could potentially touch through my work. My spiritual growth allowed me to see through the illusions the divorce culture has placed on us. I was able to detach from the labels as well as their cultural implications. I carved out my own meaning and redefined what divorce meant for me. I refused to subscribe to how culture saw it. I saw how culture operated only from two places: fear and control. I refused to live my life in its clutches.

It was only when I began to reframe the idea of divorce that things truly began to shift for me. This divorce wasn't a break from anything on the outside, it was a divorce from my own past, my own inauthenticity, my own false self, my own ego. It was really a divorce from fear and control. When I began to approach divorce as a personal declaration in my life's journey, everything fell into place. I became empowered instead of disempowered. I came into alignment with my inner truth. I entered an expansive heartfelt space of compassion, rather than blame and resentment. I wasn't angry at all. I was actually in deep reverence for all the lessons I had learned. I didn't see this as an end as much as a completion, which requires a different energy.

As I began to deconstruct all the lies about divorce, I began to ask, Does this process really need to be contentious, or can I construct a new paradigm for it? Do I need to enter fear and scarcity, or can I plug into abundance and empowerment? Does this need to be a *me versus you* experience, or can it be an experience of unified consciousness?

I knew that how I framed this process in my mind would drastically influence the state of my heart and my whole being. I first needed to enter the right consciousness. The only person I could change was myself. I kept reminding myself to focus on the highest good of all, including my husband, regardless of his emotional energy. How he behaved was not as much my focus as how I behaved. The only thing that mattered was how I chose to show up. I intuitively knew that how I showed up would reverberate in my daughter's psyche for decades to come, and therefore in her offspring for generations to follow. How I conducted myself would be the hallmark of my burgeoning consciousness as an empowered and awakened woman. Just because there were legalities or norms laid down by the culture didn't mean I needed to follow them. I chose to break free from all pressure to conduct my divorce in any way that didn't align with my essence. I made a commitment to stay in a loving space as much as possible and to keep the well-being of my family in my consciousness. I knew that if I succumbed to my ego's desire for avarice, pettiness, or competition, I would be out of alignment with my vision for my new self. No matter what, I needed to do this for myself, my new self—a woman who doesn't allow fear and ego to rule her anymore. Every step I took and every decision I made needed to be in alignment with this higher vision of myself.

If I was loyal to my essence, it wasn't because I was weak—quite the opposite. It was a declaration of my marriage to my new self to remain rooted in authenticity, away from ego. This divorce was not from my husband per se. It was about my marriage to my authentic self. Every step forward was not so much away from him as toward my truth. When I kept this vantage point in mind, I allowed the highest consciousness possible to seep through my being. This enabled me to almost float through the muck of all the form-based nonsense.

When I hired my lawyer, I told him that I was in total charge of my divorce and he was only lending me his legal advice. I told him that I would not be following traditional legal conditions but instead would be guided by what was the best for my daughter's emotional health. I informed my lawyer that if he pushed me toward decisions that would leave my husband compromised in any way, this would be unsound advice, as it would harm my daughter. If I won but my ex lost, then, ultimately, my daughter would lose, and this was unacceptable to me. I told him I would not be bullied or fearmongered by legalities or by what was considered legally fair. I told him that I would be defining these concepts for myself. Basically, I made it clear that he would be working for me and things would go as I said even if they contradicted his advice. "No conflict, no bullying, no menacing," I insisted. If he did any of these, I would fire him.

A year after the divorce, the lawyer can now see my point of view. I explain this in detail to offer women the assurance that they can indeed take charge of their choices and not feel bullied by the legal system. They can carve their own realities as much as is financially possible. The real battle isn't the legal one, it's the one between the cultural institution of divorce versus our essence.

I still remember how my hands shook uncontrollably the day I signed my first check to my lawyer. I sobbed at the loss of what was. I remembered details of my past with my ex and the good times we had experienced instead of just the bad. The vacations, the dinners, the birth of our daughter. How could I not? There were so many moments in the past twenty-five years that came rushing to my consciousness as I signed the check that I couldn't control the flood of emotions. I allowed myself to feel them. It was natural to do so. Unless I allowed the feelings to wash through me, I would not be fully processing my genuine emotions.

I was in utter fear concerning the unknown future. Yet even as fear crawled over my skin at night, I kept turning inward. I knew my fear was coming from my ego and from that which culture had indoctrinated in me. I knew I needed to go to another place in my mind, a place away from ego's lack and scarcity. Each time I turned inward, the answer was clear. This was absolutely the thing I needed to do. It was time for me to blossom on my own and find my true self outside the context of my marriage. I needed to push through my fears, which is what I did. I kept walking forward step-by-step, one foot in front of the other.

The institution of divorce advocates a 50-50 approach. This keeps both sides engaged in negotiation and, often, conflict. The decisions around who gets the piano and who gets the heirloom art piece can take eons to sort through. If one took the more expensive jewelry, the other wants to be compensated equally. Back and forth, back and forth, the couple gets mired in the battle of "form."

While this sort of battling may work in some instances, it's not always the wisest approach. Getting stuck in dividing every asset or block of time with our kids can end up creating havoc and immature fights. As long as we stay stuck in this kind of model, we actually stay betrothed to the form of things, such as pennies and furniture, instead of the formless aspect of the bigger picture—connection, harmony, and peace. It's not about who wins what, but about the greatest win for everyone. When we focus on the greatest good for all, we allow ourselves to surrender to "losing" something without necessarily seeing it as a defeat.

The end of any relationship is traumatic on many levels. It's natural to want to blame the other and fight over objects and money. These conflicts give us an illusion of control and power, two things we feel we are desperately lacking at the moment. Whatever power we feel we lose on the internal level is displaced onto our outer world. We act as if vases and dishes matter. The truth is that this is our way of scrambling for a sense of inner control and mastery. If only divorce attorneys could see that and help their clients instead of capitalizing on them, the process of divorce would proceed much differently.

Our inner void and sense of helplessness during this process lead us to don the persona of "fighter." This takes our eyes off the spiritual prize. The only way to negotiate the rough waters of a divorce is to watch how our inner powerlessness can convert us into tyrannical monsters greedy for power, creating a monster of hegemonic power on the outside. This is why we recruit divorce attorneys who are reputed to be "sharks." But things don't have to be this way at all. If we can process our inner feelings and not project them onto our partner, we can stay in our emotional lanes and allow for the process to flow without the constant stakes of egoic victories.

The truth is that the real battle for power is ultimately not an external one but an internal one. It is because the institution is set up for conflict that it thrives on our confusion and inner chaos. If lawyers were more spiritually enlightened, they would know this external fight for things is a displacement of the real fight for inner power and control. If they were truly interested in uplifting their clients, they would gently tell them it doesn't matter who gets the tea set and who gets the necklace. Neither is going to make you feel any better at the end of the day. These are false victories. The real victory lies in redeeming your inner sense of worth and empowerment. Focus on this. Lawyers don't do this because their livelihood depends on our greed and manipulation. The more we are caught up in these conflicts, the more they earn. It's up to us to realize this for ourselves. This is where we take our power back from the institution of divorce.

Not all divorce attorneys are out for capitalistic gain, of course. Some divorce attorneys have a higher consciousness and lead their clients down a more enlightened path. The point is that attorneys, priests, professors, doctors, teachers, or anyone that is the "professional" should have no emotional dominion over us. We get to choose how we steer our emotional ship. So often are we beguiled by "professionals," or "experts," even "gurus," that we lose our sense of knowing and our center. This is once again an extension of our culture's and our family's abduction of our power. So accustomed are we to losing our voice that when faced with someone who is an "authority," we readily cede our power.

In order for me to reframe my perspective about my divorce, it was pivotal for me to define what victory meant for me. What would victory look like? When I finally set out a vision for what victory would be, I aligned myself with it and was able to make clear choices. Victory for me meant that my daughter would suffer as little as possible. It was up to me to help her feel loved, validated, and secure through the divorce process. Once I was clear about this, I ensured that all my microsteps led to this vision. It meant that I would not linger over the paperwork nor fight over details.

I know that not everyone can afford to make this choice. For many, this might be the exact opposite of what they should do. Like I said before, the external manifestations of the choices we make may be different for different people. For some, fighting in court with perseverance may be the path they choose. For others, it may be a version of what I did.

What ultimately matters is not what we are doing on the outside but how we feel on the inside. At the end of the day, it's not so much about what we do or what we own but how resolved we are within ourselves. I kept reminding myself of this truth and kept asking myself, How do I feel about things? Are my choices in alignment with my authentic self? Am I operating out of fear or abundance?

The power to rewrite any aspect of our past and present lies within us. The more we honor ourselves with love and celebration of our essence, the more we will rewrite our lives with abundance and joy. As we take back all the power we have meted out to others, we can begin to align our lives according to what matters to us.

We are the scriptwriters and the narrators. We are the directors and the actors. While there are always unknown aspects of life with which we need to contend, the power to shift the scene and the storyline lies within us. We must always remember that the power to experience our world lies in ourselves. We cannot give this power away. It's our most valuable resource.

Entering the Birth Canal

For many of us, the final moments of "waking up" are terrifying, even petrifying, as we leave the old dimension of cowering fear, crippling dependence, and passive compliance. As much as living in this state is an ordeal, the idea of moving away from it is paralyzing, for no matter how treacherous our lives are, it is all we know. It is familiar, comfortable, predictable in its own mad way. Here, we might have built relationships, even married and raised a child. We might have lost ourselves a million times only to find ourselves for a few moments before being abducted by unconsciousness once again. We might have laughed and cried an ocean here. It may be the only home we know. Letting go of this life, despite its incredible challenges, is unfathomable to us, bringing its own traumas and new fears.

Despite the pain our attachments and addictions have brought us in the past, they are dear to us. We've spent decades entrenched in these patterns. They represent who we believe we are. As our old self is eviscerated, the death demands grieving. To bypass it for the sake of being "spiritually superior" is to once again fail to honor the truth of the pain we are experiencing.

As all the plans we made in our zombielike, unawakened state begin to crumble before our eyes, what was once a predictable future now morphs into a long, lonesome tunnel. We begin to realize we are dying to the old, the familiar, the predictable. All our veils are being stripped away, our masks shredded. We might walk around for days wondering how we could have spent decade after decade living a life in which we were spiritually mute, deaf, and blind. How could we have allowed ourselves to exist in such a state?

It scares us to confront the unknown. Truth comes knocking, but we are too scared to answer the door. Many of us just let it knock away till it becomes exhausted and leaves. Our entire life then becomes a stink. We fill our days with screen time, medications, and other distractions. These are preferable to opening the door of authenticity. Culture has women terrified of courting truth, let alone marrying it.

Movement into the birth canal of transformation inevitably brings regression as well as a whole lot of grief. How could it not? As one part of ourselves dies and our old skin is shed, it's natural to enter a state of mourning for what was. As we begin to speak our truth, we might begin to feel so good that to go back to deceiving ourselves feels repugnant. How can we go back once we have had a taste of heaven? The only way is forward. This inner alignment helps soothe our fears and shine the light even when there is no clear path ahead.

Leaving the old means leaving all that came with it. Many who go through this tunnel think they can take the old dynamics with them, but they quickly realize they can't. We realize we need to "adult up" and make tough choices. We can no longer be children who fantasize about having it all. It is time for us to take the fork in the road.

As we enter the process of rebirth, we mourn the familiarity and comforts our old life gave us. We might find ourselves clinging to who we were even though our old life might have brought us pain. Some of it is still near and dear to us. In my case, I was attached to the idea of being a "good Indian girl" who would never get divorced and a "good mother" who would never break up her family. My attachment to these ideas kept me in great suffering. Each time I felt the pangs of guilt within, I wanted to regress and crawl back into my old self. It took all my gumption to march forward.

My guiding light was, What is true to my authentic self? I knew deep down that as long as I followed my authentic voice with compassion and consciousness, it would all be okay. After the blood had been shed and the broken bodies buried, there would arrive a time for the resurrection of the soul. And if it was true for me, then ultimately it would be true for all.

It took me two long years of intense self-reflection and meditative practices to override the voice of my ego. It took two long years to bring my husband to a place of a modicum of acceptance and release. Mostly, it took me two long years to fully let go of the old and manifest the new.

This process taught me just how much pressure there is on women to fit into a mold and check off all the right boxes. Mothers have the pressure to stay married and keep the family together whatever the cost. But mothers are not the only ones under pressure. What about women who don't wish to get married or have children, or who want to enter lesbian, bisexual, transgender, or polyamorous relationships? What is to become of such a woman? What kind of emotional cartwheels will she need to spin in order to escape the scorn? When there is a "good" way to be and this is defined by narrow standards, living outside these lines is a perilous endeavor. Better to stay in the confines and conform.

In my own awakening, whenever my inner voice would admonish me with guilt or shame, saying "you have to," "you should," or "you cannot," I examined where it was coming from. I asked myself, What would Shefali do right now if she had no fear? What do *I* feel right now? Soon I didn't have to ask. My authentic self was no longer buried. Soon my true self and I were one. I began to live as myself.

As I unleashed my inner knowing, I used it as a beacon. It became my personal North Star. My inner voice rang with clarity. The more I listened, the more my heart opened and the more joy radiated from within me. As my daughter saw me blossom into my truer and truer self, she too let go of her attachments to what once was and allowed herself to welcome all that her new situation offered her. The dawn of a new day had finally arrived.

As you read these words, you may wonder, Am I living authentically? While it may feel like an intimidating question on many levels, the fact that you are even asking it is a turning point. When this question begins to be part of your internal dialogue, your life starts to pivot in a new direction. Like a flower that turns its head toward the light, you begin to turn your life toward this quest for authenticity. First we have the arising of the question, and then we have an organic unfolding of the path toward its answer. Just by being here, you have already begun the walk toward a new sunrise.

Part Two

~

Confronting

the

Shadow

~

~

7

The Many Faces of the Ego

The reflection in the mirror is often not a pretty sight
The crevices and cracks beneath the mask are too vivid to ignore
We try to bring others into the scene to diffuse the glare
While the fissures keep getting more ebullient
Until finally both the image in the mirror
and the mirror itself cracks.

Gear shift ahead. Now that we have explored how our fear rules us in part one, we are ready to see how we adapt to these fears.

To keep fears at bay, we don masks of the ego. These have helped us adapt and survive childhood. As we grow up, these faces of the ego become our second skin. After several decades, we wear the masks so well it's hard to tell what's false and what's true. It's only after we become aware of the masks and let them go that we can begin to shift our patterns.

The ego will not be dismantled until we begin walking toward wholeness. Our internal holes need to be replaced by a sense of wholeness, which is a feature of our authentic self. The task isn't to kill the ego, it's to heal the inner spaces where our true self failed to develop.

Although interchangeable, each of the faces of the ego has specific qualities we can learn about so that we recognize them in our lives. One facade can show up in one type of relationship, while a different situation calls forth another. When I describe the qualities of these facades, I'm seeking to understand how our psychology operates and sets up our external dynamics.

Everyone can have an opinion about their own or someone else's behavior, but it's only when we understand the root of the behavior that we can begin to connect to ourselves or another. True understanding brings about deep empathy.

The following chapters allow you, the reader, to identify yourself in its themes and scripts. You may find yourself identifying with several of them all at the same time. This is natural. As you do, keep the spotlight turned inward, asking yourself, How do I use masks to obtain validation in my life? How does my unworthiness directly employ these egoic strategies? As you begin to reflect, you will not only better understand yourself but also others in your life.

The Givers: The Victim, the Martyr, the Savior, and the Bleeding Empath

The facade of *The Giver* is one of the most common defenses our ego employs to triage "good" girls when they are in despair. When the good girl fears rejection and abandonment, she immediately deploys this facade. Placing a mask on her inner truth, she forsakes it in order to sacrifice herself for another's comfort.

This facade shows up in those women who tend to be sensitive and empathic. Their inherent blueprint is to give of themselves. Shrinking and dimming themselves for others comes naturally. When threatened in any way, they go to this default and exaggerate their foundational blueprint. This gets injected with steroids when fear enters the picture.

"Givers" are typically codependent, meaning they are highly dependent on another's validation. In fact, one could go so far as to say that their entire sense of self depends on it—so much so that without this they feel as if they don't exist.

Following are several of the masks *The Giver* wears. Identifying with any of their aspects may help you be aware of how these constellations show up in your life so that you can transcend them during moments of internal strife.

The Victim

Marilyn, age fifty-three, came to me when she was undergoing a paralysis in her growth. She wanted to quit her dead-end job but didn't know how to move forward. She knew she needed to advocate for herself either to get a better position or to look for something new.

I offered Marilyn many options for change, including becoming more confident in asking for a raise. We even practiced what she would say to her boss. We made timelines, schedules, and deadlines.

Even after four months of consistent therapy, there was no growth. She had many justifications for why she couldn't create change. No matter what solution we came up with, she invariably found a way to sabotage it. As her therapist, I remember feeling defeated. Was something wrong with my approach? When it was time for her session, I began to feel sorry for myself. Then it dawned on me. I realized that I was feeling what *she* was feeling, sorry for myself! Marilyn was playing the classic victim.

I began to replay her pattern for her. I showed her that no matter how clear the path out of her situation might be, she always had an excuse. She would tell herself, "I just have bad luck with these things. They never go well for me. I don't know if I can do this." Or she might say, "I tried to look for another job, but every time I speak to the HR departments, the people there are always so rushed. They don't seem to care about my résumé. It's like I don't matter to them."

Marilyn's body language was that of someone ten years older. She always looked harried and complained constantly. If it wasn't her work, it was her unsupportive husband or her demanding mother. Everyone and everything was at fault but her.

Once I caught on to her ego's facade, I confronted her with it. To say she was resistant is an understatement. She was downright infuriated. "You think I'm just making these things up? You are just like everyone else. Just like my husband, who doesn't even want to help me anymore. Now, neither do you! I knew you would turn out like everyone else." It was only because of my insight into how her ego was baiting me that I refused to bite. I stayed patient and compassionate, reflecting back to her each of her defenses.

Marilyn's floodgates finally burst. "I hate my job. I hate my marriage. I am miserable and don't know how I got here. I'm trying so hard to keep things afloat, but everything is falling apart." She was finally speaking straight to the gaps within herself. Her despair was now stronger than her ego's defenses.

I was able to gently show her how her ego had set all of this up so that she could play the victim. I asked:

Do you feel as if you are the "poor" one in your life and work?
Do you feel as if people take advantage of you?
Do you feel sorry for yourself and wish things were different?
Do you feel as if you are right and they are wrong?
Do you feel insulted and belittled by others?
Do you expect things from others that don't come to fruition?
Do you feel as if you are an innocent target for others' wrath?
Do you share your woes with others, expecting sympathy, and
    then feel upset when you don't get it?
Do you feel if others were different, then you would be different?

When she answered each of my questions in the affirmative, I shared that this is typically the pattern of those who see themselves as victims. The pattern is put in place in childhood as a way of keeping ourselves small.

We explored how Marilyn might have absorbed this pattern. I didn't even need to explore too deeply before she exclaimed, "My mother! She is the eternal victim. She is always the wronged one. I grew up feeling guilty for her pain." Having learned from her mother that blaming the world and being stuck in a woe-is-me pattern was a way to cope, she was unconsciously repeating this to remain stagnant.

There are millions of us women like Marilyn. Our victim consciousness keeps us mired in the lesser-than position, where we endlessly wait for the other to change or someone to rescue us so that we can be free. The irony is that nothing is ever good enough. We are so unaccustomed to joy that we are resistant to it even when it stares us in the face. So hardwired are we to expect despair that we automatically assume the worst, thereby fulfilling our prophecy that nothing good will ever happen to us.

This victim consciousness is a tricky thing and hard to shatter. It offers the perfect refuge from our fear of not being worthy or loved. Victims stay stuck in this mindset so they don't have to be accountable for how their lives have worked out. They are afraid to change because of even the slightest possibility that things won't go well.

Before we move forward, I must clarify that there is indeed such a thing as a victim. For example, one can be a victim of rape, or brutality, or racism. This is not what I am alluding to here at all. I am speaking to a victim *consciousness* where we stay mired in a way of thinking that locks us in the lesser-than position. Here, no matter what our present reality, we harbor a persistent sense of feeling attacked or "done to" by another. A victim *consciousness* is more a mentality than a position one is put in through an act of emotional or physical violence.

Beginning with her boss, Marilyn saw how she was using others to play out her internal script. She took off her blinders, which allowed her to now see him as a human with limitations like herself. Once she released her role of being "done to," she was able to request a raise and a new job description.

When we "play" the victim, we may hear our self-righteous tone and feel a sense of helplessness. Thoughts abound such as,

"I cannot believe this happened to me. After all I sacrificed and gave up, I could never imagine I would be treated in this manner." A victim is always the "poor" one. She is always being taken advantage of by someone.

In order to transform out of a victim consciousness, we need to take hold of the reins and advocate for ourselves. Feelings of blame and helplessness need to be transformed into action. Each day that a victim awakens with a renewed sense of purpose and direction, she takes one small step closer toward change.

When the victim wakes up to the fact that no one placed her in the position of disadvantage, and that it was her subconscious choice, she may at first feel disillusioned. To realize that you yourself are the cause of your own "poor me" status is a sobering encounter with reality. To discover your presumption that you had no choice is a total fallacy is disorienting. You might feel as if your entire world is crumbling.

As you realize that you always have a choice about how you show up, you move away from silently suffering in a victim consciousness to a vociferous self-advocate. You begin to choose empowerment over subservience, slowly leaving behind those who were addicted to your self-suppression. If you are able to brave your way through this fiery transition, your victim consciousness will become victor consciousness, unlocking the invisible shackles that have bound you your entire life.

The Martyr

Sasha comes to mind when I describe the martyr complex. Sasha is a driven corporate lawyer who is also a mom, a dutiful daughter who takes care of her invalid father, wife to a busy CEO, and a staunch environmentalist who gives at least twenty-five pro bono hours to charities each month. She is always on the move. The only reason she even agreed to come for therapy is because Anna, one of her daughters, was suffering from anxiety in her first year of middle school.

At first Anna was dropped off at sessions with me by their nanny and only occasionally by Sasha. It took a lot for me to cajole Sasha to come for a few sessions. During the sessions, she apologized profusely for her lack of presence.

I could identify with Sasha and had an immediate liking for her. Accomplished and competent, she was a woman who simply didn't know how to say no—the classic martyr. When I told her this, she immediately began to laugh. Clever and witty, she said, "I knew you were tough and direct, but I didn't know just how much. You have blown my whole cover to smithereens."

We had a good laugh—a laugh shared by two women who are comfortable acknowledging their neurosis. I explained to her how she had set up every moment of her life to be in the service of something outside of herself, sacrificing her own well-being and even that of her children.

To help her clarify the many ways this role played itself out in her life, I asked her:

Do you see your role in labels such as Mother Teresa or
    some heroic saint figure?
Do you walk into spaces and situations and take over the whole
    show?
Do you typically endure your hard work through noble
    suffering and silence?
Do you feel burned out by all you have put on your shoulders?
Do you feel resentful because you feel taken for granted?

She said a resounding yes to all of it.

"It's so hard for me to complain," she replied. "But on the other hand, I feel that if I don't complain, no one will give a damn about me. No one ever asks how I'm doing or how I'm feeling. They always take it for granted that I'm okay. Yes, I am okay—and I'm happy giving to everyone else. But I also feel exhausted and at times used, so I typically just sigh and moan in silent protest."

Once Sasha saw that I was onto her deeper patterns, she began to come regularly for therapy. We uncovered what lay beneath her martyr complex. She had grown up with an older sister who had a chronic disease. She watched her parents obsess over her sibling and run themselves to the ground giving her 24/7 care. Sasha was always made to feel guilty for being healthy and normal. She reminisced, "If I ever complained about normal kid problems, they treated me with contempt, calling me ungrateful. I felt guilty being me. I grew up so upset that I wasn't the ill one that I literally envied my sister."

There it was—her version of not being good enough. She truly felt she was bad for being who she was. The only way to exorcise this badness from herself was to do extra good, presenting herself as the heroine. This was the source of her need to do everything for everyone, including the animals and the earth itself. She was determined to make up for not being "the broken child."

In one of our sessions, Sasha broke down. "I was never even noticed as a child. I didn't even exist. I was only recognized if I could be of help to my parents." As soon as Sasha said these words, a quiet descended on her. She then whispered, "I am resentful of everyone in my life, actually. I have given them my entire existence and they keep taking and taking. I resent them, just like I resented my sister. Oh my goodness, I have literally re-created my entire childhood, haven't I?"

As we become aware of our feelings and how our ego has created a false persona, the inner holes that have been yearning to be filled by our true self come into the light and we can move toward wholeness.

It was time for Sasha to grieve the losses of her childhood so she could begin to integrate this loss instead of hiding from it. She cried for the rest of the session. Gone was the competent put-together attorney. In her place was a shuddering, defenseless little girl. Without her ego, she was raw and honest. Sasha was finally coming back home to the little girl she left on the sidewalk of her childhood.

Once we see what the true needs of the neglected child are, we can go on a quest to meet them. Sasha realized that instead of sublimating her inner needs in service to others, she needed to transform them into service for herself. She now had to begin the joyous path of reparenting herself. All the attention her parents had given her sister, and she in turn bequeathed to others, she now needed to lavish on herself. As she put herself first, she slowly began to shed the unnecessary duties and obligations she had placed on herself in order to meet others' needs. She began to let go of her instinct to overcompensate for everyone's shortcomings and slowly began to nurture herself. She finally arrived at a place of comfort where the others' discomfort did not stab her heart anymore. What a relief this was indeed.

Martyrs often complain of body pain and neurological stress. They are literally burdening their nervous system by grossly neglecting their own self-care. The antidote to the martyr complex is self-honor. They need to place themselves in the position to receive attention, compassion, and service. All they give to others, they need to give to themselves. This sounds selfish and narcissistic, but it's exactly what martyrs need.

As the martyr turns the spotlight toward her own self, she is bound to feel selfish. At first, she will not even know how to do it. The first step in self-honor is for her to declutter her life from all that's extraneous. This itself involves an arduous letting go. As she sheds the weight of others' expectations, she will slowly begin to breathe more freely. She will soon discover her own authority, releasing the need to obtain validation from others.

Part of this letting go is firing herself from all the extra roles she's taken on, such as being on the boards of nonprofits, parent-teacher associations, and hospital charities. As the need to be a martyr evaporates, in her place there will be a woman who is unafraid to be unapologetically flawed, ordinary, and most of all human.

The Savior

I don't think I know of a single therapist who doesn't suffer from this face of the ego. I am sure most people in the helping professions have these qualities.

I spent my early twenties with a burning desire to help others. While this was a good motivation and propelled me to do many a kind thing, I went to the extreme. I didn't just want to help, I wanted to rescue. Not just rescue but cure. If I passed a bus stop in my car, I fought the urge to stop and offer someone a ride with little thought for my own plans. Or if someone was in financial duress, I wanted to step in and take care of all their woes for them.

I finally had to ask myself, Did they ask for help? The answer was no. My desire to excessively invade boundaries to help people hardly ever came from the other. It was something I made up in my head. This naturally led me to inquire, Where is this need to save coming from?

I soon came to see how this was a mask for something deeper. My "savior" had a darker side. Yes, it was loving and kind, but its extreme nature showed me that it was also fulfilling an inner longing. I had so much empathy and compassion for the pain of others that I wanted to ease their struggles. On the other hand, I was so uncomfortable with their tears that I was actually trying to save myself from the pain of seeing them suffer.

My longing was for many things:

My giving allowed me to feel significant and useful, valid, and worthy.
My giving allowed me to not confront my own pain about the other's pain.
My giving allowed me to ward off the discomfort of tolerating the unknown.
My giving allowed me to feel superior and competent, powerful, and in control.

My giving attracted broken people to me, allowing me to
   continue this cycle.
My giving allowed others to depend on me, which gave me a
   sense of power.
My giving allowed me to not learn to be a receiver.
My giving meant I could distract myself from my own self-care.

Those of us who are saviors deflect the loss of our authentic self
by focusing on others. This allows us to maintain a persona of
goodness, even superiority, which is our way of compensating for
feeling inferior.

I still remember an early supervisory session when I was in my
twenties. I was telling my supervisor how I went over time with my
client by an entire hour because I was helping her with her broken
car. This wasn't a one-off situation in which the client had unex-
pectedly found herself in an emergency. This was someone who repeatedly set herself up to be dependent on others. The problem she
had with the car was one she had known she needed to fix.

When I told my supervisor that I offered to drive the client home,
he nearly fell out of his chair. He looked at me with an odd mix of in-
credulity and pity. I knew then that I had done something drastically
wrong. Whereas I thought I was being compassionate, he explained
how I was operating out of a savior complex. I was fascinated. I had
never heard of such a thing. He showed me how I had fused myself
with my client and totally identified with her ongoing struggles as
if they were my own. There were zero boundaries between her and
myself. He then lovingly showed me how I was actually setting her
up to be dependent on me, crippling her instead of empowering her.

This was my introduction to my savior complex. I thought this
was it—I learned about it and now I could conquer it. Little did I
realize that it would take decades to overcome and was actually
part of a larger problem. As I continued my journey into wholeness, I began to realize how insidious this identification with the
savior was and how I needed to detach from it. This is a hard thing

for us in the helping professions, as it is for most women, especially the more maternal and nurturing ones. One of the reasons we enter these spaces of healing and motherhood is that we have caring hearts and giving personalities. To put boundaries around these traits doesn't come naturally, but if we don't, our ego's defenses can grow so large that we imagine ourselves messiahs, here to heal others.

Many therapists have such delusions, as do many religious leaders who call themselves all sorts of labels, such as "guru" or a derivative of God such as "Reverend." Once I got in touch with my own savior complex and saw it for its hidden narcissism, I was appalled. Where had I developed this delusional idea that my influence over another was so great? How had I overestimated myself so egregiously?

I was able to let go of my savior complex once I understood how I was hurting my clients by taking away their own resourcefulness and the growing pains involved in their own development. I was robbing others of their own authentic struggles and snatching away their power to find solutions. Once I saw this clearly, I knew that I needed to immediately annihilate notions of saving anyone.

Ashley, my forty-seven-year-old client, was hell-bent on saving her children from feeling any strife or pain. She first came to me because both her children were violating her wishes in the home and wreaking havoc. Not only did they rarely help around the house, they used her credit card without permission. Ashley was at her wits' end when she came to see me. "I try so hard to do everything for them. I can't understand why they treat me so badly," she confided.

I asked her, "Why do you work so hard for them? What are you trying to achieve?"

"I just feel so bad for them," she replied. "Their father left us when they were young. Since then, I've carried the guilt of raising them without a male figure in their lives. Once I realized how traumatized they were when he abandoned them, I've tried hard to make it up to them, but nothing I do ever works."

I empathized with Ashley. She was coming from a loving place, as all of us are. I explained that her desire to over-give wasn't because this is what her children truly needed. The desire to over-give came from something deep within her, a guilt she experienced that was unbearable. Her regret and remorse at what her ex-husband had caused them to endure was something she couldn't let go of. As a way of compensating, she tried to save her children from their pain. Little did she realize that she was actually saving herself.

Now, after years of giving them everything they wished for, but setting none of the boundaries they needed, they were running amuck. I showed her how she had actually ended up doing them a disservice. She had made them believe that they lived in a world where their wishes would always be granted and they would always be saved by others. As a result, they treated her as the wish granter and their personal concierge. What mattered to her was irrelevant to them.

When I showed Ashley the pattern she had been living out, her jaw dropped. She was shocked at how she had been blinded by her own guilt, and how this had been the driver of her actions. With this realization, she immediately felt even more guilt! Her identity had been so wrapped up in her savior image that to learn she was self-centered came as a jolt.

Some facades of the ego go undetected because culture encourages them, especially in the case of women. We get stroked and endorsed for these facades. It's only when we begin to self-destruct that we are prepared to crawl out from under them. The ultimate reality is that we operate under these facades because we are afraid to show our true selves. We have learned over eons that these facades of the ego are the way to receive validation, which is why we continue to be enslaved.

The antidote to the savior complex is to learn to tolerate suffering, starting with our own. Most saviors create this persona as a way to avoid sitting with their pain. The idea that the other is in pain, particularly if caused by the savior, is so overwhelming that she seeks to eliminate it. She figures that if she rids the other of their pain, they won't have to experience the feelings around it themselves. The savior feels a sense of competence by rushing to another's rescue. The "fixing" of another gives her focus and redirection. The only way out of this pattern is to realize that there is no one on the outside to save or fix. We cannot do this even for our children or our loved ones, which is a bitter pill to swallow. The only person we can do this for is ourselves.

When the savior realizes the other's pain is necessary, and even vital, for them to awaken to their own true self, she is able to turn to her own pain and the many ways she has avoided the discomfort it brings. She needs to go through a detox and resist the temptation to solve other people's problems.

Instead of turning toward others, she now begins to turn inward. She begins to ask, How can I heal myself from within? In doing so, she slowly begins to take care of her inner pain. She allows herself to cry where before she never did. She begins to tolerate her own pain better, and through this inches toward growth. As she sees the power in this and understands how this act of turning inward could have the same effect on another's life, she sees how her saviorship was preventing others from going within and addressing their own pain. Instead of rushing to save others from confronting their pain, she teaches them to invite it in with open arms.

The Bleeding Empath

When I was young, I attended a Catholic girls' school in Mumbai, India. Even though I was raised without a religion, this was the school my parents chose to send me to as it was one of the better ones in our neighborhood. One of the ways Catholicism was spread in India during British colonialism was through the education system. Eager for their children to be westernized, many parents forsook the typical Indian schools for these Catholic schools even when their children weren't being raised Catholic at home.

When it was time for morning prayer before a test or a final exam, I noticed all the Catholic girls stood up to pray with great fervor to Jesus. They furrowed their brows, clenched their hands in prayer, and gently rocked back and forth. They seemed desperate to make a last-ditch plea to Jesus to redeem them during the test. My young eyes took it all in. Rumor had it that their parents often whipped them with belts if they came home with poor grades. My heart bled for them.

I made a plan. I would give them my quota of blessings from God. Not being raised with any religion per se, I didn't really have a personal connection to any deity. I hoped that wouldn't work against me. I stood up and prayed to their God, and all the gods I could think of, begging them to give the other girls good grades. I bartered with them that they could give me a bad grade and award some of my better grades to them. My parents didn't put pressure on me to do well. I hoped that the gods would understand and take care of my friends. I did this from first to third grade.

I remember this because it shows how my bleeding empathy started young. By the age of seven, I was helping nurse an elderly, sick man in our building. I helped his wife change the bedsheets and lay out his clothes. I visited him every single day till he got better. I was the only kid in my neighborhood who would leave the playground early and stop by his house to play his favorite card games. No one needed to tell me to do this. I did it because it was my nature. My mother is a classic bleeding empath. She taught me through her example to raise my own empathy to an extreme. I learned to care deeply for other people. It's little wonder I became a psychologist. My capacity for empathy allows my clients to feel held, validated, and understood, which is part of the process of becoming whole. But the same empathy led me to blur the lines between self and other, with their pain becoming my pain, and their story mine.

While being giving, intuitive, and caring are certainly good traits, like all facades, they can be taken to an extreme where we ignore aspects of our authentic self. I began to see how I locked myself into this role as others soon expected me to be there for them against all odds. When I wasn't available, they were upset with me, as if I had violated their birthright of having me at their beck and call. My attachment to this role made me feel excessively guilty. It was my mission to be there for others through their struggles despite the cost to my own self-care. It was only when I realized that I was in the "role" of empath that I could begin extricating myself from it. I made a list of the typical traits that made me veer toward excessive empathy:

> The capacity to feel the other's pain to a deep degree
> The capacity for compassion for others' circumstances
> The desire to alleviate the other's suffering
> The willingness to help others at any cost
> The inability to hold clear and consistent boundaries
> The inability to ask for help and receive it with openness
> The incapacity to clearly state my needs without guilt
> The tendency to feel hurt when the other doesn't appreciate
>   or validate me
> The hardship in saying no and facing conflict
> The inability to tolerate conflict and tension
> The desire to have others need and depend on me
> The tendency to be super giving, super helpful.

Once I listed my patterns, I was able to observe them with a certain degree of objectivity. When I did so, I began to see how I set up my relationships the way I did.

Empaths in general have an overwhelming desire to be validated as the "good" one. Their giving often veers into excessive self-sacrifice. If the giving includes receiving, then it isn't considered giving at all. There is a hidden conditionality the empath is often not in touch with. When the other changes for the better, the empath feels great about herself. When there is no change, the empath feels despondent, belittled, and resentful.

One of the main shadow aspects of extreme empathy is that it typically goes hand in hand with dismal boundaries. Empaths find it hard to say no to the ones who need them. Empaths excuse all bad behavior as stemming from the other's pain. Because they deeply feel the other's pain, it's virtually impossible for them to separate the bad behavior from the pain from which it stems. As a result, they never hold the one they are helping accountable. Suffering from the fallout of destructive behavior, they prefer to attach themselves to the role of "the understanding one."

The empath's desire to give to an excessive level comes from her own inner lack. Her identity depends on how much another is dependent on her. In this way, she harbors a shadow side of narcissism where she enjoys being needed and in demand. This is why empaths typically enter intimate relationships with predatory narcissists. Both fill their empty holes by depending on and feeding off the other.

For an empath to understand herself, she needs to undergo a systematic deconstruction of her patterns. This means turning the spotlight on her cocreation of reality. The first thing she needs to be aware of is how she has been giving of herself as a way of obtaining love and worth. Her inability to say no doesn't come from a lack of desire to say no, necessarily, but from a fear of conflict and abandonment. Until she is able to get to the source of these core fears, the empath will not be able to construct the boundaries she needs to thrive.

For years, I have listened to women blaming others, especially their partner or ex if they are unhappy with them. "It was his fault. He was so mean. He was such a jerk." Of course, they are always justified in their outrage. They were, after all, "the good one." That's how their ego set it all up. Perhaps they really wanted to say, "No, no more! I won't allow you to treat me this way. I am too worthy for this relationship," but were always too terrified. So instead of stepping into their courage, they allowed the other to continue their mistreatment so that they could continue feeling like they were the more "understanding one."

Since we "good women" find it intolerable to be "the bitch," we continue to be what our ego has trained us to be—compassionate, kind, understanding, bigger than the other who just dumped their stuff on us. So another moment of ill-treatment slips by, another boundary violation goes unnoticed. Our inner resentment grows stronger, we feel shame, we blame ourselves or the other, and the cycle continues.

This kind of deconstructing is extremely challenging. It's painful for the empath to come to a place where she realizes that the reason her feet keep getting stepped on is because she places her feet in the direct path of the other's shoes. As with all awakening, this realization comes as a shock.

The antidote to bleeding empathy is a healthy dose of self-worth and self-care. When the empath is in touch with her inner sense of self, she will naturally execute clear and consistent boundaries. Through boundaries, she can elicit her wonderful qualities for love and nurturance while being careful not to enable the other to be inconsiderate of her needs. In order for her to have empowered boundaries, it's imperative that she surrenders her own attachment to the idea of being "the good one." Once she can let go of her own unconscious agenda, she will be able to realize the importance of sacred boundaries.

Boundaries often get a bad rap because of the fear that they can create disconnection. This isn't the intention of boundaries. When created from a place of inner alignment, boundaries create healthy relationships. They hold the capacity to teach both parties how to enter self-reliance.

An empath begins to heal herself when she changes her internal script. Where before she might have valued excessive giving as the only way to function in relationships, she now begins to learn how to receive. As she realizes her worth and that she is deserving of receiving, her ability to create healthy boundaries grows. These boundaries will be viewed as sacred containers within which her beautiful heart can breathe freely and joyously.

I can honestly say that I have pieces of each of these Giver archetypes within me. Perhaps you feel the same way as well—as if these different faces are melting into one another. This is natural. After all, our psyche is not compartmentalized in defined shapes. Keep absorbing the insights and journal about those facades that fit you the most. Soon it will be clear how your primary ego facade shows up, and you will understand what strategies you most use when you are in a state of lack.

~

8

The Controllers

The Perfectionist, the Helicopter, the Tyrant, and the Shield

Controllers are highly anxious people who convert their anxiety into controlling their environment so that they can feel in charge and competent. They disguise themselves as achievers in the case of the perfectionist, worrying caretakers in the case of the helicopter, dominating control freaks in the case of the tyrant, and an impenetrable rigidity in the case of the shield.

Givers want to show the world how good they are, whereas controllers want to show the world how competent they are. A giver cannot bear to be seen as self-absorbed, and the controller cannot bear to be seen as a failure. Both are ruled by a morbid unconscious desire to answer their burning internal question, Am I good enough? This is the question all ego archetypes ask themselves.

Controllers, as their label implies, constantly control their life situations, relationships, and possible outcomes. They quell their anxiety that they aren't good enough by channeling this energy into controlling everything in their sight—more housecleaning, more cooking, more exercise, more hovering over their children, more preparing for x or y, more work, more ambition, more makeup, more clothes, more of a meteoric rise in their profession, more control and bossiness over others. These are people who go to the extreme in whatever they are doing and attempt to become master micromanagers.

Controllers cannot sit still. Their inner anxiety is so high that they must relieve the pressure by doing, doing, and more doing. They are often exhausting to be around and cause a flurry of anxiety in their wake. Let's explore their different masks and see if any of their aspects resonate with you.

The Perfectionist

While a sense of achievement and excellence are healthy and even vital for daily living, perfectionists go way beyond what's healthy. They seek to be meticulously and exaggeratedly overprepared. Ever vigilant for any possible error, they go above and beyond what's required, taking charge of every contingency and ruling out every chance of failure.

This desire to be perfect can make a pendulum swing to the other side, with the person giving up before they even try. Morbidly afraid of failing, they are paralyzed to try at all lest they aren't successful. Although this pattern is harder to detect and is often labeled laziness, it's worth remembering that passivity and performance avoidance can be a disguised manifestation of the same plague, that of perfectionism.

The driving force behind the perfectionist's behavior is the avoidance of failure. The prospect of not being a success or underachieving is so unbearable that every measure is taken to avoid it. The outcome of any venture is tied to how the person feels about who they are. They are willing to go to battle for the outcome of such a venture because they know that if they do well, they will feel amazing. Conversely, if they do badly, they will feel lousy. The inner pendulum is tethered to the external outcome. The anxiety over being considered mediocre or just average crushes their inner self.

Tia is a perfectionist on steroids. She is a beautiful, skinny woman in her fifties. She has been used to adulation where her beauty is concerned, so much so that she is nonchalant about it. None of this matters. All that matters is that she is not a size zero. She looks at herself in the mirror and doesn't see the vivacious beauty that others see. Instead she sees what she considers are her drooping chin and saggy jaw. She points out wrinkles and creases as if they are ripping her skin apart. She complains constantly about the way her inner thighs touch when she moves. As a result, Tia has pursued every type of cosmetic surgery out there. You name it, and she has done it. From Botox to liposuction to face-lifts to fillers and more, she has tried it all. She has relentlessly pursued every new body-improvement invention and still feels dissatisfied and discontented.

Tia has been coming to me for therapy for the past year. No matter how much I have tried to counsel her, her self-loathing is constant. If I compliment her, I inevitably hear something like, "Thank you, but . . ." Where perfectionists are concerned, self-acceptance and self-celebration are distant qualities.

Tia isn't alone in this. I have seen innumerable friends and colleagues plagued by the burden of perfectionism. It shows in overpreparation and in its converse, paralysis. So burdened are perfectionists with the desire to control every single unknown that they either spend years preparing for unseen disasters or they simply stop in their tracks and enter a comatose state.

The perfectionist is tortured from within by a staunch and severe inner critic that constantly goads them. Their inner voice sounds like this:

You have to constantly do and perform in order to feel good.
You need to outdo your last performance and do better each
    time.
You need to either excel or give up—average is unacceptable.
You cannot trust anyone to do the job because they might mess
    it up.
You should double-check everything and conduct risk
    assessments.
You should do more, try harder.
You need to focus on the 1 percent that went wrong or that
    might go wrong.

You don't want to start new projects unless you are assured of
   success.
You need to be highly critical of yourself when you don't reach
   the outcome you desire.
When things don't go as planned, this means you are
   incompetent and unworthy.

Mika is a professional speaker and is present at the many con-
ferences I attend. She typically paces backstage rehearsing her
material over and over. She confesses to me that she chooses her
outfits months in advance and hires speaking coaches to perfect
her pitch. "There is nothing wrong with this desire to be excellent," I say to her, "but there's a vast distinction between striving
to be the best version of yourself versus striving for perfection."
One drives us to constantly learn and grow. The other drives us to
"perfectionitis." While the former is adaptive and useful, the latter
is maladaptive and dysfunctional. Two very different motivations,
two very different ways of being.

Perfectionism gone awry turns into "perfectionitis," a near-
mental illness. When we take our desire for excellence to a paranoid
level, we allow it to control us, robbing us of our joy. Joy can only
burst forth from a state of presence and spontaneity, which are undermined by our judgmental thoughts.

I know that Mika suffers from "perfectionitis" because while
she is preparing and pacing up and down, she is also downright
terrified. She has her notes, her PowerPoint, and the Xanax bottle
from which she takes two tablets at breakfast. She collapses like
this prior to every talk, telling me, "I am so scared that I'll forget
what I am supposed to say or do that I get worked up into a tizzy."

Life doesn't come with a guarantee of success each and every
time, which the perfectionist expects. Only when the perfectionist
learns to go within and sit with the painful anxieties around rejection and failure can she learn to tolerate the inherent groundlessness of life. When she begins to cull a sense of inner worth from her
own natural state of being, without needing to do a single thing,

she will let go of her delusions of control and settle into the fact that a life best lived is one that surrenders to its lack of control.

Perfectionists will shift from within when they realize that a mistake or a failure is not only inevitable but downright necessary for improvement. Until then, they will view these as plagues to be avoided. Only through deep self-love can perfectionists let go of their delusional standards and release their shame around failure.

The Helicopter

Elisha was adamant that her daughter needed to attend a college that was within a two-hour drive from where they lived. Her daughter Cheryl wanted to go to the other coast, which meant they were in a constant battle. The daughter stomped out of a therapy session one day stating she felt smothered around her mother.

Elisha was devastated and wanted to run after her daughter. I had to get up and lead her back to her chair. "You cannot run after her. She is not five years old. She is almost an adult. What are you worried about?"

Elisha replied, "I am worried she will hurt herself. She is so mad at me, I don't know what she'll do. I feel I need to be there to make sure nothing bad happens."

Elisha is the classic helicopter parent. She is overly attentive to her children's needs and overly involved in every aspect of their lives. She treats them no differently than when they were toddlers. In her eyes, they are still defenseless and immature.

In my individual sessions with Cheryl, she confessed she capitulates to her mother because she is afraid of her mother's rages. Now that it was time to go to college, Cheryl was anxious she wouldn't be able to go to the college of her choice.

Elisha refused to see anything wrong in her style of parenting. She refused to own that she was being driven by anxiety, which had nothing to do with her daughter. Not unlike the hundreds of other helicopter and hovering parents I have met in my practice, such parents trend toward overprotecting their children, morphing into their children's 24/7 butler, concierge, chauffeur, and private maid service.

This ego facade isn't restricted to parents. It runs across many relationships and takes on many shades. Their extreme desire for control shows in a few different ways:

Overpossession—the other is seen as a direct extension of the self

Overprotection—the other is treated as a precious object to be safeguarded

Overscheduling—life is micromanaged and scheduled to the minute

Overcriticism—finding blame with everyone and everything

Overmanagement—the other's life is managed as if it were one's own

Overinvolvement—boundaries are crossed, and the other's life is taken over

The helicopter parent is driven by an intense anxiety concerning her powerlessness, which is displaced onto others. Unable to tolerate her inner state, she projects this intense energy outward.

In her fifties, Stella gave birth to Janet after many failed in vitro fertilization (IVF) treatments. Naturally, she treated this miracle baby with kid gloves. She booked an appointment with me because her husband forced her to. "He thinks I am going to ruin Janet's life with my craziness," she told me.

Going on to describe "her craziness" she confessed, "I am terrified of her falling and hurting herself, so I don't let her come out into the backyard with me because there are steps where she might fall. I make her wear a helmet at home because I don't want her hitting her head against the wall. I don't let her out of my sight at the playground." She went on to give me a dozen examples of how terrified she was of her child getting hurt. On the one hand, she came across as vigilant while, on the other, she was the uber-helicopter mom.

We began to excavate her intense desire for control. She had undergone nine IVF treatments over the past seventeen or so years. It's hard to judge someone who has gone to so much effort, with all the angst and turmoil involved. Little wonder that, now she had achieved her goal, she felt like she needed to protect this treasure.

Obsessed with her mission to be the best mom possible, her identification with her child ruled her life. She wanted to preserve her identity as the most caring mother possible and to prove to herself that all the years of struggle were worth it. If Janet were to be hurt or sent to the hospital, in Stella's eyes, she would have failed as a mother. So desirous was she of competence that she rendered herself helpless.

Rather than going within to uncover the source of her insecurity, she overzealously protected her child. By making sure nothing ever happened to Janet, she would be exempt from having to deal with her own sense of incompetence as a mom.

Many of the women I grew up around were helicopters. I have an aunt who cannot sit still. She simply cannot. She always has to arrange and rearrange things, cleaning and tidying. As a kid, watching her made me feel dizzy. Her anxieties make it unbearable for her to relax and simply be. Unless she is constantly doing, she is afraid something terrible will happen.

Most helicopters don't even see themselves as controlling. They see themselves as caring. This is how their ego lures them into maintaining their behavior. If a woman has a view of herself as attentive and supportive, how does she shed this role? The only time she will is when she can admit that her excessive caring is driven by her own anxieties and, consequently, her own self-protection. When she sees that she is doing damage to the ones she loves, she may perhaps stop. Admission of her desire to control is key.

Helicopters have to learn how to release their desire to control life. In short, they need to learn the art of surrender. When they understand that life is inherently chaotic and impermanent no matter how hard they try to control it, they may learn to stop their incessant doing and start being present. Only when they are able to accept the utter futility of control will they able to release and surrender to the is-ness of life.

Trusting the is-ness of life is not easy for any of us, let alone the helicopter. She has learned to ward off feelings of vulnerability by micromanaging her environment, especially her loved ones. At first, this backing off will seem strange and cumbersome. Funnily enough, doing less may feel extremely arduous to her. As she slowly learns to back off, she will learn to channel this energy back to herself. She will release the others in her life to their unique destiny and fully embrace her own.

The Passive-Aggressive Tyrant

This persona is a supersize combo-pack of the giver and controller rolled into one. She is the chameleon commander on steroids.

Typically the woman who exhibits this facade is a pleaser. She is passive, sweet, compliant, docile, adaptable, and easygoing. She is happy to please the others in her life and typically puts up little or no resistance to changes in plans. Where this becomes a problem is that she will please at all costs, mostly to avoid her own true feelings because she is afraid of conflict. Any form of conflict scares her. In order to control the level of conflict around her, she will bend over backward to make the other's needs more important than her own. She feels a tremendous inner pressure to pull everything off with a smile.

So how does this lovely persona morph into a raging, aggressive tempest? It happens when she bends backward so far that she breaks. For example, she wants the house spick-and-span for a party. She wants the guests to be happy and well fed. She wants everyone to get the best service. So she slaves away all day. Her husband and children don't have the same aspiration. They are happy with the house disorganized. Here is where all hell breaks loose

and she becomes a resentful tyrant, tired and frustrated, screaming at her family for not caring as much as she does.

Many a mother will completely relate to this. I know I do. We
spend every moment taking care of our children, our house, and
our loved ones, saying yes all day long, maintaining our cool. We
are unaware of how this impacts us in subtle ways. We don't realize
how exhausted we are by all this giving. We stretch our emotions
and bury our fatigue, blur our boundaries and hide our tears—until
we break. So ignorant are we of our unmet needs that we combust
and our rage bursts forth. Of course, we release it on the wrong
targets, often our children, which breeds guilt.

Once we combust, we are mortified. We cannot believe we just
did this after an entire day of holding it in and giving. We sense
we've ruined it all. This is the fate of the passive-aggressive tempest. She is stuck in a cycle of pleasing others at all costs but doesn't
pay attention to when her own boundaries have been overstepped.

The cycle she falls into has these elements:

She says yes to all the requests made of her without discretion
     until she is exhausted and rageful.
She doesn't speak up about her needs until she burns out and
     breaks down.
She ignores her self-care to the point of developing chronic
     illness.
She controls others and micromanages them through guilt.

The truth is, we don't want to say yes to every request. We don't
want to work so hard. Nor do we want to feel guilty for saying no.
We don't want to control others, yet we keep doing so.

My client Sheena comes to mind. She began her first session with
me by crying her eyes out. She confided that she needed to take an
anger management course because she was losing her mind with
her children. "They are good girls, but I expect them to be perfect. I
literally yell at them all day long. I expect them to be little soldiers."

With two children under the age of six, Sheena was an over-achiever. She cooked fresh homemade meals every single day, cleaned her house, and also managed all the bookkeeping and finances for her husband's company, together with all the home bills and repairs. The sad part? All she saw were her own failures as a mother. She didn't realize that she was trying to achieve an unrealistic expectation of who a mother should be.

"Why are you feeling all this pressure?" I asked.

"My husband expects the sheets to be ironed and everything to be immaculate," she confided. "His mother made every meal fresh and at home, so he expects this from me." She described her husband with a degree of reverence, then revealed, "My husband thinks I'm not organized enough or hardworking enough. He thinks I should accomplish more and should be putting more effort into my motherhood and wifehood."

This is where the problem lay. Sheena was trying to pander to her husband's unusually high standard of how a house should be run. In her efforts to meet his standard, she was ruining her children's childhood by enlisting them as minions in her army.

When Sheena saw what she was doing, she was horrified. She admitted, "I want to tell him to back off, but I'm afraid to. I'm scared we will have a conflict, and I hate that. Conflict terrifies me. I also want to be his ideal of the perfect woman, like he sees his mother."

Sheena revealed how her father had abandoned them when she was little. She was raised by a single mother who worked a few jobs to make ends meet. She learned early to be the perfect little girl so that she never stressed her mom. The only problem now is that she cannot be perfect enough. No matter how much she does, it's still not enough for her exacting and perfectionistic husband.

The antidote for pleasers is to "fire" the bosses they are trying to please. Every pleaser is trying to please someone they have put on a pedestal. The pleaser wants to do all she can to gain favor in the eyes of this person, so much so that she will enlist everyone around her to help. When I showed Sheena how absolutely amazing she already was, and how she had been falsely worshipping her husband, her eyes flew open. We traced the reason for this obsequiousness to her fear that her husband would abandon her like her father did. Somewhere in Sheena's psyche lay the deeply embedded notion that had she been a better daughter, her father would never have gone. This is why she went all out in her attempt to be super amazing in her marriage, unconsciously warding off the possibility that her husband might leave.

I explained, "You have made your husband your boss. He didn't ask to be your boss. Sure, he is bossy, but that doesn't mean he gets to be your boss. You gave him that position. Fire him! This unequal dynamic is creating havoc within you, which you then take out on your children. You are the boss of your own life. If your husband isn't happy, he can make the changes he needs to make. You cannot contour your every cell to make him happy. That is his own job. Fire him right now!"

Sheena began to see how she had given her husband the role of her father, boss, and approver. She *needed* him to approve of her. The more she needed this, the more she succumbed to his insane expectations. If she began to embody her own "boss-dom," she could send him back into his own lane and flourish in her own.

This individuation process is key in enmeshed relationships where one is dependent on the other's approval. Sheena was still unconsciously waiting for daddy's approval, as well as fearing daddy's abandonment. As she began to grieve her past and integrate her losses in her adult world, she took her husband off the pedestal. By normalizing him as a flawed human being, she was able to create boundaries and turn her attention where it needed to be—not on the dishes and homemade pizza dough but on the joy of her children.

Sheena snapped out of the cycle of passive-aggressive tyrant. She knew she was risking the approval of those who were addicted to controlling her, which was daunting. But she realized that such a loss, if it came, would be okay. After all, she was gaining a whole new boss, friend, and lover—herself.

The antidote here is one thing only: enlisting oneself as one's own boss and validator. As long as we try to receive validation from the outside, we will be in constant inner misalignment. We will seesaw back and forth until we snap from within. The tight rope of inauthenticity will break one day and all hell will break loose. As with the other ego facades, the more we are honest with ourselves, the less likely are we to combust and burn.

The Shield

This woman is easy to spot because she stands out from the crowd. As rare as she is, we have all met at least one of her kind in our lives, and it is almost impossible to forget her. This is a woman who appears always in control, always in charge. Smooth, cool, unemotional, tough, rational, and independent, this woman will not allow you to see her out of sorts. She is hell-bent on always having it together.

Typically, such an alpha woman learned early that in order to gain control in life, she needed to step into her masculinity big time. This persona was probably born out of having experienced trauma and abuse as a child. It makes sense for such a girl to develop a shield to protect herself from abuse. Part of this shield requires her to be impenetrable, and part of being impenetrable requires not being vulnerable. Invulnerability requires a person to be nonemotional, strong, and independent. In short, it requires her to ditch her feminine side.

This girl grew up with the belief that she needed to conquer her world in order to feel powerful. She became overachieving, overzealous, and overdriven, typically climbing to the top of whatever she is doing. You may find her as the leader of organizations, political parties, or movements. We have much to thank her for, but we cannot forget that her defense comes at a price in terms of her well-being.

Kylie embodied this archetype perfectly. There is almost nothing she cannot do. "I had to be the boy and the girl in my family. I was expected to be just as good at sports as baking, be top of my class in science, and excel at sewing and other traditionally girly things." Now, at fifty-three, she is an accomplished psychiatrist, author, and concert violinist. Her Achilles' heel? Relationships. She has the hardest time and experiences her greatest challenges around relationships.

"I just cannot tolerate any sort of emotional drama," Kylie opined. "This is when I shut down. It feels chaotic and threatening to me. Emotions signal danger. I cannot show my own or allow others to show theirs."

Kylie's past few relationships ended abruptly. When a few problems showed up and her partner of the moment acted in an emotional way, she shut down and avoided him. It's as if she expected her partners to be just like her, rational at all times and almost detached.

We began to explore Kylie's aversion to emotional displays. True to form, the road took us back to when she was six and lived her life with a strict, alcoholic father prone to rages. In a fit of anger, he told her that he wished she had never been born and confessed he had always wanted a son. What hurt her more than her father's displays of rage was the fact that her mother never stepped in to protect her. Kylie could trace his underlying resentment of her birth to how he always pushed her to play rough-and-tumble sports, something she didn't relish, and how he always teased her if she cried. He would yell at her when she showed any signs of weakness. Many times, he hit her with a belt. At times she would cry for her mom, who never seemed to hear her pleas for help. Constantly taunted, bullied, and abused by her father, and neglected by her mother, she learned to develop a tough exterior and slowly watched her true self wither away.

I explained that this "shield" she had developed was protective during childhood, but instead of helping her now, it weakened her connection with others. We outlined the specific ways she had set up her personality so that she could clearly identify her patterns:

Stoic and unemotional
Rational, detached, and logical in arguments
On the serious and quiet side, unable to let loose
Overachieving, oversuccessful, and overorganized
Is a walking Google of sorts—keeps data and facts at her
    fingertips
Avoids emotional movies or conversations
Is the person others turn to for disaster control

The description hit the nail on its head, and Kylie laughed at herself—a rare occurrence. She quickly began to see how she had created this persona both to protect against her father's rages and also to become the son he always wanted.

Women who wear this protective armor often like solitude and quiet. They don't like people in their emotional or physical space. It's easy to neglect them and forget that they may be hurting. Their impenetrable exterior, coupled with their natural competence, makes it hard to connect with them. They make people feel as if it's best to leave them alone. What these women miss out on is human connection.

It took Kylie a few months to shift. She was so uncomfortable with showing up as herself that she almost had to be retrained to speak a whole new language. She had to learn to tune into herself on a regular basis. I had to coach her by asking, "What are you feeling now?" Then I would ask again, "And now?" I had to repeatedly inquire, "And now?" She was so accustomed to going into her head, using pure rationality, that she had no idea how to look inward. However, she was slowly able to do it and became better at allowing people into her inner life.

The antidote to those who wear such a tough exterior mask is to train them to begin to feel their feelings without intellectualizing them. With baby steps, such women need to incorporate the heart, not just the mind. They need to use words like "I feel" instead of "I think." They need to learn that feelings are not a threat or a weakness, just another form of communication. If anything, being able to show up with their feelings is a strength.

So conditioned are these women to believe that emotions are a defect that they severely deprecate themselves for harboring feelings. Their growth comes in learning to trust that they can handle their feelings by taking greater risks, meeting more people, and trying new things, thereby becoming a more whole person.

9

The Takers

The Diva, the Princess, and the Child

Are you feeling as if you are every single one of these descriptions? Your overwhelm is understandable. As versatile beings, we exhibit different parts of ourselves at different times. However, once you read about all the different personas, you will recognize that there are only a couple that predominate in each of us.

So who are the takers? Unlike the givers and controllers, takers operate out of a lack of self-governance. Divorced from their internal power, they glom on to others and extract their resources as their lifeline. Takers depend on others to do things for them and to provide emotional sustenance.

Much like the narcissist who has learned to be self-absorbed to the point of not recognizing the needs of others, the takers, too, have learned to protect themselves by entering a position of self-absorption. In a passive-aggressive helpless way, they begin to depend on those around them. Let's look at some of the common manifestations of the takers.

The Diva

The diva is one who believes she has earned the right to boss people around and have things her way. She believes she is better than others, period. Because of this superiority complex, she has fooled herself into believing that others are there to serve her. She believes she is entitled to this service.

Typically, though not always, a diva is someone with a few accolades under her belt who has had a taste of being a "star." Because she has identified herself with being a star, she believes she needs to be treated as one. She expects undivided attention, unlimited praise, and favors from all.

I have typically seen this energy in those who have achieved some rank or celebrity status, or some position of social influence and prestige. But I have also seen it in families where one person assumes the hierarchical head position and uses this status to boss others around. So thirsty are they for validation that they believe in their social persona, expecting their audience or family to fawn over them. Of course, when this attention is short lived, they typically crash with a nervous breakdown or addictions.

It isn't uncommon for women who have accomplished something that gives them status in society to put on the airs of a diva. On the one hand, it might certainly be an achievement that they have broken ceilings to get where they are, but this certainly doesn't warrant lording it over others. This is the ego's way of keeping us tethered to the validation of others.

Stephanie had been chosen to play a supporting role in a Broadway show and was over the moon. This was her lifelong dream. I saw her morph from a simple girl into a starlet. While an embodiment of one's power is always positive, it turns sour when the diva persona overtakes the person's essence.

This is what happened to Stephanie. Before long she was incessantly complaining to me about her coworkers. They were too amateur and pedestrian for her liking. Even the director was unprofessional. She wanted her peers to recognize her as someone important. When they didn't, she experienced a narcissistic rage. She felt entitled to better treatment than she was getting and was severely stung when she didn't receive it.

She came to me because she had just received a harsh and negative review for her performance, which devastated her. She was unable to reconcile this feedback and bounce back to normal. She was thinking of quitting acting altogether. Her need to be superior to others was so great that this was trumping her love for acting. When I broke down elements of the diva energy for her, she was in shock. These are some of the aspects I highlighted:

The need to be the star of attention
The need to receive only positive validation
Negative feedback is a plague
The need to be perceived as better than anyone else
The need to be treated with kid gloves

When Stephanie saw how she was playing the role of the diva, she was embarrassed. When I asked her to remember a time in childhood where she had last been treated like a diva, she recalled when she was in third grade and had starred in her elementary school play. She replayed details of how special she felt, especially how proud her mother had been. Her own mother was a well-known local actress whom Stephanie had always wanted to emulate. Being in the spotlight felt wonderful to little Stephanie—she had craved that moment all her life. Alas, Stephanie was never cast in a lead role, which has always made her feel unworthy. This Broadway show was the closest to the main part she had received since third grade.

Thrust in the limelight, Stephanie finally felt more worthy and secure. She didn't realize that she was employing the persona of the diva in order to create a hierarchy between herself and those around her. Her need for power was stemming from her inner lack of it. So thirsty was she for validation that she just couldn't tolerate anything negative being said of her.

As a public person myself, I have seen quite a few of my contemporaries embody the diva energy. They feel entitled to a different level of treatment once they are somewhat famous and feel miffed when they don't receive it. So starved have they been for this sort of validation that they are insatiable for its nectar and enraged when this is denied.

Diva energy should not be mistaken for power since it doesn't manifest from an awakened heart but from a feeling of emptiness and lack. Divas attempt to take from others what was denied them in their younger years.

Diva energy is common among parents, where mothers sometimes step on children, lording over them a power that they could never exercise in their own childhoods. I observe that mothers-in-law can sometimes exercise this same energy over their daughters-in-law.

With a culture that is intensely starstruck and willing to project all sorts of halo effects onto those in the limelight, it's easy to get swept away by thinking you are indeed the wind, moon, sun, and stars. When I found myself enamored by the praise I was receiving when I first started out as a public figure, I knew I had to do some deep spiritual work. I began to ask myself, Why does it matter so much to me what other people think of me? Am I that empty within?

When we are devoid of an inner connection to our worth, it's easy to get swayed by the opinions of others. It's as if we need others to construct our sense of self. This is why most of those who achieve stardom too early in life, before they have found who they truly are, are destroyed in the public arena. Swayed by the number of likes and unlikes they receive, their sense of themselves is constantly called into question.

Because a large part of my work is in the public eye, I had to learn to distance myself from the court of public opinion. When I do a Facebook live or a talk on stage, I inevitably get thousands of reactions that range from what I wore and how I looked to what I said and whether they agreed or not. It's important for me to listen to feedback and grow from it, but it's dangerous to become prey to the capricious projections of others.

It was only when I fully divested myself from all sorts of opinions, even the positive, that I liberated myself. The positive and negative were only the projections of strangers who had nothing to do with my personal reality. If they found me competent, it wasn't because I was necessarily so, but because they were in accord with what I was saying. If they found me totally idiotic, perhaps it's because I clashed with their deeply held beliefs. The key is to detach from both the lovely comments as well as the negative ones.

Diva energy stems from deep insecurity. When we are in this kind of energy, we are competitive and negative toward others. We are filled with a harsh inner critic that is mercilessly scathing. Only when the diva is willing to go within and be honest about her inner demons will she be able to break this pattern. She will need to stop the pretense and begin to tell the truth of how she really feels inside—crummy, unworthy, and small. When she is in touch with this inner space, her mask can drop. A beautiful thing happens next. People begin to see her true self and they relate to her more than ever. As she receives genuine connection from others, she realizes she no longer needs the facade of the diva. Connection trumps them both.

When we revert back to our quiet internal place, we find there is nothing to be a diva about. The truth is that we are always worthy, diva or not, and until we can access this deeper truth we will forever be foraging for approval.

The Princess

The princess employs the facade of one who refuses to step into her power. She is developmentally stuck in her preteens or teens, rebellious and entitled, but refusing to grow up. Entering adulthood feels daunting to her, so she waits for others to step in and take care of things for her. She feels entitled to be handed opportunities and expects to be pampered. She doesn't necessarily lord it over others like the diva—she simply waits and passively expects.

Debbie had been seeing me for a few months when she revealed that she was miserable in her marriage. Although smart, she reported never fully pursuing anything too deeply. "I dabbled in everything, from sports to my academics. Nothing gripped my attention." Life happened, children were born, and Debbie stalled on pursuing a profession. It was now a distant dream. In her marriage, Debbie complained that there wasn't much intimacy or emotional connection. Her husband, a successful doctor, was hardly ever home. She complained that he neglected her and that he always put his career or their kids before her. She felt listless and bored. I suggested that she look for a job or volunteer somewhere to keep herself fulfilled.

Weeks passed and her complaining continued. She wanted more passion and purpose in her life yet didn't take a single concrete action toward either. She and her husband were in constant negotiation around how much she could spend. Debbie never seemed happy with his budget. I suggested that she could earn her own money and become independent of her husband.

Much like the victim, Debbie felt slighted. But unlike the victim, she also harbored a sort of a passive entitlement in her stance. "Why can't he just give me an unlimited budget? He has plenty of money. I want to remodel the pool house, but he refused. I hate when he's stingy like that. I wish he was like other husbands who are generous with their wives."

Wanting another to take care of us symbolizes the princess complex. We believe our right is to be nurtured, protected, and provided for. It doesn't occur to us that we need to make equal or similar contributions to our own life, let alone that of others.

When I dove deeper into Debbie's psyche to explore exactly why she didn't want to get a job, her excuses ranged from:

I've never had a real job.
I don't know whether I am work material.
I will need at least another year.

She had the same reply to every suggestion I made: "I don't know." The reason she didn't know is because she didn't need to know. There was someone else, in this case her husband, who was doing the knowing for her.

Helplessness and stagnation are the hallmark of the princess. She isn't evil or even manipulative, just exasperatingly self-absorbed. She doesn't feel as if she has the power to execute actions she needs to take. Her default is to ask for help even when she can complete things on her own. So ingrained is her sense of helplessness that others in her life just naturally pick up the loose ends.

Debbie continued to wait for her husband to increase her budget and for him to approve the renovations on the pool house. She also continued to wait for the ideal job to fall into her lap. All through her waiting, she kept expecting things to change. When I pointed out that things couldn't just change on their own, she was at a loss. "What should I do?" she asked. I knew better than to answer a question I had already answered innumerable times. I now recognized her question as part of her persona of helplessness.

When people ask too many questions before starting a project such as, "How will I do this?" or "What should I do now?" they at first sound genuine and earnest. It's only after having answered them a few dozen times that we catch on to the fact that this is a habit of passive helplessness.

Once I saw the energetic intention behind Debbie's confusion and recognized it as an intentional obstinacy and paralysis, I stopped rushing in to rescue her with suggestions and strategies. I recognized that she was terrified of taking action. More than this, she was afraid of growing up and becoming autonomous. It was much easier for her to wait on others to take the risks she was afraid to take. In this way, she could blame the other and keep herself off the hook. By telling herself that things didn't work out because of someone else, or because she tried hard but nothing really panned out, she could preserve her identity of being faultless.

When I outlined Debbie's persona to her, she was quiet at first and then burst into tears. She said that she didn't realize she was so transparent and didn't even know that her ways of being were conditioned. She just thought that this was who she was. These are some of the patterns I helped Debbie identify:

Defaulting to helplessness and not knowing how to do things
Terror of entering adulthood and being responsible
Purchasing attention and love through helplessness
Protecting the psyche from failure by being passive
A sense of entitlement and anger when help isn't given

When we traced Debbie's issues to her past, we uncovered how she grew up with an overachieving elder brother. She remembers how he got all the attention, and how she felt neglected and alone. The only way she used to get the family's attention was when she fell sick or something bad happened to her. She learned early to fall into states of passivity as a way to draw her family's attention to her.

The princess is scared of failing, being rejected, and—more than this—feeling as if she is a worthless fraud. The only antidote to this complex is to hit rock bottom. Most people only change when they are at the dead end of their resources and absolutely nothing works anymore. For this to occur, everyone in the princess's life needs to cease their collusion, since she is upheld by her enablers. Once her enablers stop allowing her to stay in a state of passivity, she will have no choice but to become resourceful.

I still remember telling one of my clients, who was a classic princess, that I simply couldn't help her anymore. She was devastated. I gently told her that not rescuing her was actually the best thing I could do for her. If I kept allowing her to depend on me, I would do her a disservice. She tried to make me feel guilty by crying, "How could you leave me?" I knew that her helplessness came from her ego and not her true self, which was courageous and powerful. I told her to make certain changes in her life and only come back once those were complete. I am still waiting for her call. I don't take this personally. I understand the power of the ego's ways, which can keep us stuck in patterns interminably.

Debbie began to heal only when she reached a complete stand-still. Her husband refused to change and rescue her. He even asked her for a divorce. Her kids were away at college and beyond. There was nowhere for her to turn. This was her rock-bottom experience. The first thing she did was get a part-time job, which eventually morphed into full time. She resisted the hard work at first, but as she began to save money, this boosted her self-confidence and gave her a sense of autonomy. Her self-confidence eventually turned into self-worth. I was honored to watch her transformation from passive princess to full-grown adult.

For the princess to want to change herself, she will need to go cold turkey and detox from her dependency on others. She will need to become an adult who is in charge of her life. Once she sits in the driver's seat of her destiny, she will find that it wasn't such a scary proposition after all. She will notice with a smile that the view from the front window is verdant and inviting.

The Child

The child lives in a bubble of comfort, complacency, naivete, denial, and an ephemeral sense of hope and optimism. She is the eternal Peter Pan. Afraid to grow up and face reality, she is typically a woman who feels comfortable being in exactly the same town and job, if she works at all, or following a predictable and comfortable routine.

The child doesn't enjoy change, conflict, or upheaval. She would rather keep the status quo and be relatively miserable than create a change that holds the possibility of bliss. Her security is more important than her authenticity. As a result, she enters a docile, conciliatory position of servility that allows her to keep strife and conflict at bay. She holds on to childish fantasies and keeps waiting for them to manifest, all the while not doing much to bring them about. She appears cheerful and positive, but this is because she lives in an unrealistic version of a reality that will never come to be.

Denial and avoidance are the hallmarks of the child. I find this persona most often played out by women who are in relationships with men who do not treat them as well as they should, and yet these women conjure a fairy tale around their situation that allows them to maintain the status quo. Or if they are working, they have fantasies about their bosses or coworkers, saying things like, "I hope one day he will walk into work and realize all that I have done for him as his assistant." They may tell themselves that one day the married man they are with will leave his wife and "come be with me. Until then, I know that he really wants to do it but just can't." They live in the world of "one day," like a child who says, "One day I will be the president of the United States," or "One day I will be an astronaut."

I can still remember my first session with Melody. She entered the room in a long, pale-yellow dress looking frail and worn. Her knuckles were twisted together in a knot, white with trepidation. "I think my husband is having an affair," she said. "I'm not sure, but I see signs that indicate this. It isn't the first time." When I tried to explore how she had dealt with his infidelities, she said, "I didn't say anything. I just thought it was a one-off. Then it kept happening and I hoped it would stop. I was just in shock that he would do such a thing, so I treated it as an aberration and not the norm. Now it is happening again and I cannot believe I am here in the same place I was almost a decade ago."

Melody had never directly confronted her husband with any of these truths. She preferred to stay quiet so that she didn't rock the boat. When I asked Melody how she wanted to proceed this time, she said, "I am just going to do what I always do and wait for the storm to pass. It's got to pass over, right? I know my husband doesn't mean to lie to me. If he's lying, it isn't going to last forever. I am going to focus on the positive and let him do what boys do. After all, whose relationship is perfect?"

Within moments, Melody was able to switch out of her despondency into cheerful optimism. It was fascinating to watch. What happened to all her feelings from a few minutes earlier? I then understood what was happening to her. When Melody confronted the truth, she felt enormous inner chaos, disillusionment, and pain. It was almost too much to bear. As soon as her inner child felt the pangs of deep emotions, her ego jumped in to the rescue and masked her pain with the persona of the child. With her mask firmly placed on her face, everything changed. She went from an adult confronting the discrepancies of her disturbing reality to a child who lived in a fantasy world where nothing was wrong.

The child allowed Melody to continue being optimistic without changing her life. It allowed her to ignore the cognitive dissonance she was feeling and move into a Pollyanna state of oblivion and cheer. It was much easier for her to be protected behind this persona than to confront the painful truth of her marriage. It was only when I helped her see the ways her ego did this that she was able to shift out of her patterns. I outlined some of her behaviors to help her identify these patterns:

Stays inactive and passive in decision making

Stays paralyzed about taking action so others are forced to take it for her

Unable to tolerate pain and bypasses it to achieve cheerfulness

Great denial about the painful truths about her life

Insistence of stating she is happy even when authentic expression is not present

Lack of insight or awareness into her own or others' true feelings or pain

Stays superficial with herself and others

Doesn't like to probe into the deeper reality of her life or life in general

Avoids conflict by ignoring her authentic feelings and acts conciliatory

Those who employ the facade of the child learn early on that life's chaos is too threatening, requiring too many daring moves. Those who use this mask keep their head buried in the sand. It's much safer and predictable. All that matters is that they are protected from the pain of having to venture out of their little matchbox to confront the unknowns of life.

At the core of this persona is a wounded little girl who is bewildered by all the chaos in her life. When Melody was seven years old, her parents divorced. She said that her life changed overnight and nothing was the same anymore. No one stepped in to rescue her from her overwhelming emotions or to soothe her confusions. She remembers regressing back to an earlier age when things were happier and calmer. She began to suck her thumb and wet her bed. This brought about more anger from her parents. Despite this, she clung to her innocence and has maintained this childlike persona ever since. It is her protection that keeps her cocooned in safety and warmth. Her feelings were so scary, she vowed never to feel them again. This is why she loves to wear the mask of the child. It envelops her with joy, optimism, and hope—all of which keep her delusion in place.

The antidote to Melody's child complex is a harsh detox from the denial strategies she has adapted all these years, and a bald-faced confrontation with the truth. She already knows the truth; she is just pretending she doesn't because it's much easier to play the game of "not knowing." This way there is no one to confront, no conflict to be endured, and no changes that need to be made.

If Melody wants to evolve, she will need to take her child mask off and stand naked before the mirror of her actual life. She will need to see herself under the glaring light of awareness. As she begins to confront her life as it truly is and not as she wishes it to be, she will touch her inner resilience. She will notice that she is indeed strong and brave. Mostly, she will realize that she can stomach change and that it is to her benefit to do so. She will begin to embrace more and more change and leave behind the pall of an inauthentic fear-ridden life. As she does, her naivete will be replaced by a relentless ardor for the truth.

When the archetype of the child is at its extreme, the woman embodies the doll complex. She becomes infinitely pliable and accommodating, ready to be her owner's toy. Like a doll, this woman serves the other at the extreme sacrifice of herself. Such a persona is typically undertaken under conditions of severe emotional neglect and abuse. The doll succumbs to the will and whims of the other, whom she deems more powerful. In order to step out of this, she needs to wake up to her own voice and dare to use it. Although risky and perhaps dangerous, once she begins to execute her free will, she can break free. The victims of cult crimes and those involved in cases like the Jeffrey Epstein case are typically women with the doll complex. These are women who have long been forced to abandon any sense of personhood or autonomy which leads to their belief that their very existence is to be of service—even if this involves abuse—to others.

Releasing the Ego

It's important to remember that we are nuanced creatures and can be many things at once. My attempts to provide a classification of the faces of our ego is done with the awareness that we are far too complex to categorize. Moreover, our ego can take on many personas at the same time, with us playing first one role and then another. There are no hard-and-fast rules when it comes to our psyche. We flow with the present moment, asking ourselves what version of our ego is playing a role right now. Instead of judging and predicting our ego, we choose to stay present.

Once we are awakened to the various ways our ego plays itself out, we can stop wasting energy on the outer world and turn our energy inward by asking ourselves which wound from our past is being activated and causing us to feel fear. As we go beneath the protection our ego provides, we are able to understand why we felt the need for protection in the first place. We typically go back to early childhood fears of not being good enough and not feeling seen, loved, or validated. As we realize the ego was only protecting the fears of our childhood, we begin to have gratitude for it. We also realize that the task of reparenting ourselves lies with us. It's time for us to be the mothers and fathers to ourselves, the ones we always wanted but never had.

The ego only thrives in the shadow of our unconsciousness. As more of our inner world comes to light under the glare of consciousness, the more the ego fades. So the path to releasing the ego is to know our true self. This is where all the answers lie.

Part Three

BACK TO NATURE

Disclaimer: I fully believe that every one of us has a right to embrace our own identification regarding sexual orientation and the lifestyle that best suits us. Every woman's and man's experience should be honored for what it is, whether they identify with their biological identity or not.

In this chapter, I speak mostly to cisgendered individuals because I am deconstructing some core phenomenon that cuts across the broader demographics of this group. While I am speaking in traditional terms of sex and gender, I do not mean to exclude lesbian, gay, bisexual experiences, or those of trans men and women, nonbinary, gender-fluid, or intersexual individuals. I am sure I am excluding some, but it is not my intention. There is something to learn here no matter how we identify in terms of gender.

10

Nature's Design of Our Body

Like a masterpiece, we are infinitely immaculate
Like clockwork, we are unfathomably precise
Like a puzzle, we are profoundly complex
Like an oasis, we are boundlessly replenishing
Like the universe itself, we are unbridled, eternal, and free.

In my daughter's teen years, we often talked about her sexuality. She bemoaned how the boys she knew were emotionally immature or just interested in "hooking up." She talked about how many of her girlfriends felt the pressure to have sex and how she didn't feel ready. At times she asked me questions about sex and often shared her fears and dilemmas.

Each time we talked about sex, I breathed a sigh of relief that she felt comfortable doing so. I certainly didn't feel free to do this with my mother. There was no talk of sex, or even my feelings about it. I was just supposed to figure it out, and my mother would have preferred it was something I didn't engage in—except, of course, when trying to have a family.

Growing up, the message I received was that sex is bad. Not just bad but disgusting. If we engaged in it, we were slutty and immoral. This never fit in with my personal moral code. I just couldn't get it. If it was so bad, why was it the only way we could have kids? The taboos against it didn't make any sense to me.

A large part of our awakening journey is to entertain a renewed understanding of ourselves at the foundational layer of our biology and our body. This requires us to go to the core of what makes us male and female. We ask, How does my sex influence my psychology? We candidly enter a dialogue about our body, our sex, and our sexuality to create an awareness of how these influence us.

Nature made it simple. Most of us are born male or female. This is our sex. Our sex is not necessarily our gender. Our gender identity is both culturally and personally constructed. While for most, our sex is inherent with our birth, our gender identity is finessed over time through our psychological interactions with our family and our circumstances.

There is no definitive phenomenon known as "woman" or "man." The only objective reality is *our* femaleness and *our* maleness. This is our foundational nature, and while it can be relatively altered through modern medicine, hormones, or surgery, it is still at the core of who we were born as.

As we awaken, it's important to be aware of how nature, in the form of biology, shaped our bodies and designed us to perform the functions we do. Key questions to gain insight into as women are, What does it mean to be a female? How does having a vagina, breasts, and a predominance of female hormones affect us? How did culture capitalize on aspects of our biology and maraud it for its own patriarchal convenience? It is only when we understand our female and male nature from a biopsychological perspective that we begin to better understand ourselves as women and men.

While males and females are equal in that we are both entitled to the same rights to dignity and liberty, we are unequal in how nature constructed us. We don't have equal shapes or strength. Our biological roles are not equal. There are wild differences between us that need to be understood, and doing so will go a long way toward helping us understand one another more deeply.

How Nature Set Women Up to Nurture

A woman's body is designed to give of herself. Through this natural nurturing comes an effortless attuning to others. We are the quintessential community builders and gatherers of the tribe. It's the way of the female *tao*.

Because of her biology and how nature set her body up, a female holds within her the power of nurture. This giving nature is what culture has abused for its own advantage. When we are not consciously awakened to how culture does this, we can give of ourselves to the point of self-oblivion.

Let's take a look at how our body is set up for us to be givers. Consider the ways in which our bodies are exquisitely designed to bear children. Whether one chooses to enter motherhood or not is not the point. The fact remains that our biological architecture is set up for birthing. Consider also how our womb creates space for our burgeoning unborn child—our belly stretches to accommodate and contain the child, and our breasts know to grow and hold the milk on which our infants will suckle. This design is nothing short of miraculous.

During my own foray into motherhood, I remember marveling at how my breasts knew to lactate when my newborn needed sustenance. Where before my breasts had been the objects of beauty and sexuality, they elevated themselves to the sacred purpose of feeding my daughter. Appreciating my connection with nature, I was in awe at how my body simply knew what to do without any prodding. It was the first time I saw myself as an animal. I was, in essence, a vehicle for nature to replenish itself. I didn't feel diminished by this awareness. I felt exalted. I saw myself as one with the lioness, the female chimpanzee, and the hen. Just like their bodies give and serve their offspring, I was designed by nature to serve. I saw myself as life-sustaining, powerful, and capable. I was one with all sentient beings. I was one with the earth. She and I were of the same soil, one that blossomed, nurtured, and regenerated itself.

Although biology designed the woman to be a giver, culture reshaped her to give of herself to the point at which she loses what little sense of herself may have survived childhood. Culture drew our blueprint as a stifling mandate. Knowing the difference between the legacies of biology versus culture is the key to our awakening.

Culture realized we would be prone to give to others. Instead of allowing us to feel power in this, it undermined our capacity to feel this power. In knowing that women will accommodate and nurture, culture took advantage of our capacity to contour ourselves.

So how do we honor that which comes naturally to us without losing ourselves? How do we give and take without abandoning ourselves? Unless we are awakened to the fact that culture's imposition on our natural biological qualities has taken us down a destructive path, we will stay dormant, passive, and oppressed.

Nature wanted us to know who we are in a manner that *empowers* instead of *devours*. Awakening involves becoming aware of the difference between what's real and natural to us, and what's conditioned.

Nature didn't intend for us to lose ourselves. Nature wants women to claim the whole of who we are. This is why she gives us the option to be mothers but doesn't punish us if we choose not to be. Nature stays neutral, accepting that there are natural checks and balances in how species advance. Some proliferate greatly, and others don't. There is no shame or judgment. It just is the way it is. Culture, however, isn't so neutral. Culture suggests that adult women who are not mothers feel some degree of embarrassment, if not downright shame and ostracism. These emotions come from attachments to how culture demands we live our life. Nature, on the other hand, realizes that everyone is simply not the same and cannot be expected to be. Culture shames diversity while nature celebrates and exalts it.

Awareness of our biology is the fountainhead of all other understanding since it engenders our capacity to nurture, caretake, be empathic, and be sexual. If we are to understand ourselves psychologically, culturally, and spiritually, we must understand our biology and how it primes us to be subjugated by patriarchy.

Owning Our Vagina

Mysterious and complex, the vagina is positioned by nature in a protected and hidden connecting point between our thighs. If you look at its design, it's not unlike the bud within the folding petals of a flower—in this case the vulva covers it ever so gently. Intricately layered, the vagina itself is obscured from view as if nature evolved it to be so because of its vulnerability.

In its design, our vagina holds the capacity to be the receiver of the man's penis and the portal for the birth of the next generation. It's passive in that it's the receiver, and yet active in that it's vital for the birth of our children. In its dual role, it entertains the dance of inaction and action, receiving and giving, pulling and pushing. This dance comes naturally to us. In the past, this quality was valued by the tribal communities we lived within, where we women held places of high status and leadership. It is only in our modern-day patriarchy that we are isolated from one another and abused for our instinct to give rather than elevated for it.

Just because the vagina is hidden from sight doesn't mean it needs to be ignored and its existence denied. Nature never taught us to avoid our vagina—modern-day culture did. In modern times, we have been increasingly taught to reject our sexuality, conditioned to believe we are "bad" if we act upon our instincts. A woman's first indoctrination in this is when she is taught to avoid her vagina.

I had been brought up to believe that the vagina is a "no touch zone." We are "bad" girls if we are in tune with our sexual desire. By being denied a celebratory approach to our sexuality, we fail to connect to our own body, let alone take charge of our own pleasure. If we feel ashamed to see, touch, or feel our vagina, how can we ever hope to be fully comfortable with another human touching us?

We have disowned our power partly because we are disconnected from the power we house between our thighs. Most women
I know are disconnected from their vagina. Few of us have cultivated an intimate relationship with it. We have been told that to do
so is, essentially, to be a whore.

Do you remember your mother having a conversation with
you about the pleasures and pain of sex? Did she help you get ac-
quainted with your vagina and teach you that you can take your
sexual prowess in your own hands and learn to pleasure yourself? I
certainly don't remember any such conversations with my mother.
It was only later that I discovered all that had lain undiscovered
and took my sexuality in my own hands.

If a woman is never taught to celebrate her vagina, how is she to
know what brings her pleasure? How can she guide her lover to fulfill her? We need to be the one to guide him or her, showing them
how we like to be touched and pleasured. To do so doesn't make
us slutty or whorish. Conditioning has taught us that only "those"
women put their sexuality out there.

It's one thing to deny our sexuality as it pertains to another
human being, but quite another to be taught to avoid a part of
our body because it's associated with sex. Both involve denial
and suppression of something intrinsic and natural to us, but the
latter involves rejection of something that is a part of our body.
When we are taught to eschew a part of our body as if it doesn't
exist, we subconsciously believe it's a "bad" part of us. In this
renunciation of a core part of ourselves, a disconnect happens
within us that subtly pervades all aspects of life.

The vagina is the birthplace of all human life and the source
of our sexual empowerment. To ignore its many gifts is a trav-
esty. Getting in touch with the bounty of our vagina is to reclaim
our identity as sexual beings, something culture is desperately
against. We need to understand that a woman who takes charge
of her sexual empowerment is no longer dependent on a man, except for his capacity to help her bear children. Once she takes the

power of her vagina back, she is declaring her emancipation from the clutches of the patriarchy. This is a woman to be reckoned with. To exalt her vagina and what it epitomizes is to awaken a female renaissance.

Women have been conditioned to believe that the vagina's only purpose is to be a canvas of pleasure for another—most typically a man's sexual enjoyment. This is how the vagina gains its legitimacy. Such a belief is the source of our suppression. By seeing ourselves as only able to offer pleasure to another, we hand over the keys of our sexual liberation and allow ourselves to be minimized by a patriarchy that thrives on our suppression.

Imagine if we took this pleasure into our own hands and began to own our sexual desire and our climax? When we are able to lovingly bring ourselves to a climax, we enter into an empowered sovereignty. With this focus on the self, we light ourselves up and shine, no longer dependent on the men or another in our lives. We become firmly implanted in our own being. Dependence on a man becomes more for procreation. Pleasure would be delightful as well but more optional.

The way to sexual connectivity and liberation begins with owning our vagina. The vagina isn't merely an opening in our body. It isn't something "down there" that we need to hide beneath well-ironed skirts and daintily crossed legs. It's the birthplace of life itself. Since there is no life without the vagina, we hold within our body our future generations. Everything about it has been brought into being not only for the gestation of life but also for our pleasure. It's only when we understand the purpose of the vagina that we comprehend who we are, not only on a biological level but also psychologically, culturally, and emotionally.

When we understand how the vagina holds within it the clues to both our enslavement and our emancipation, we fully own our journey through life. To awaken means to claim power over every part of ourselves. Not power over others, but the power enshrined in our own truth.

From Subjugation to Empowerment

In her opening of herself through the opening in her body, a woman holds the power to elevate her own and her partner's sexual experience. The more she opens, the more she can dance, play with, and enjoy her vagina, offering great pleasure to the partner with whom she engages. Again, it is through this very opening that she is her most vulnerable, subject to a male's aggressive subjugation. There are no secure doors to her vagina, making her prey to a male's unwanted advances should he choose to enter her. Therefore, she must guard herself with extra protection. Much to their chagrin, every parent instinctively knows this about their daughter. She may even protest about her brother's freedoms, but she will be shushed by her parents who know that a girl is forever at risk in a way their sons will never be.

The vagina has tremendous power to give and release pleasure. The emancipated woman understands this power and chooses whom she gives it to wisely. When she exercises this choice with great discretion and discernment, she moves from subjugation to empowerment.

Unless we awaken in a deliberate and conscious way to our own orgasmic potential, we will continue to lie in service to the other, relatively unfulfilled and at a loss as to why. The woman who discovers her "warrior" side learns that her desire to serve another must be born out of her desire to serve *herself*. When she learns that her first allegiance is to her own truth, and only then to the truth of others, she shifts the paradigm in her favor. Now she can do both, adhering to her natural biological design as a nurturer and caretaker, while focusing on her own growth as a fully autonomous being who has needs and desires of her own.

When conception occurs through its own intricate interplay of domino effects, women are the ones given the sacred responsibility of nurturing the growing child. Our food becomes its food. Our blood becomes one with our child. Our body grows to accommodate the other, sometimes more than one. Expanding to nurture the needs of another is built into our architecture.

With childbirth, we move into a new dance, irrevocably intertwined with another. Those nine months of togetherness in the womb alter who we are. The sooner we bury the person we used to be and embrace the mother we are now, the less our trauma. Gestation months allow us to mourn our old identity and embrace our new one.

It is through our embrace of the mothering aspects of our biopsychologies that we truly have an opportunity to move away from culture's subjugation and rise into our empowerment. When we come into awareness of our absolutely mind-blowing potential to house, birth, and grow our children, we come into awareness of our power. Once we see how our body adapts and transforms itself to meet the needs of our children, we fall into synchrony with the natural power of the universe. We see ourselves as the earth and the ocean—a home, a garden, a sanctuary. Resonating with all in the universe that births life, we begin to see that nature made us to be divine. Only culture has maligned our minds and abused our bodies in such a drastic way that it has obliterated our connection to this divine power. The awakened woman reclaims what nature intended for her and, in doing so, frees her sisters and daughters to do the same.

Housed within us all, mothers and nonmothers alike, is an intuitive and wise knowing of our mothering powers. It is this knowing that is the key to our capacity to tend to our young with care and dedication. Once we touch upon this knowing within ourselves, we can perhaps harness it in other areas of life. Just as our body morphs into flourishing fields for our young, so we can morph into this for ourselves. Even when a woman doesn't birth children, she is still very much a mother, whether to her friends, the elderly, her pets, other children, or to her own inner self.

It cannot be reiterated enough that all women hold the mothering principle within them. We are always bearing this potential—whether biologically or socially. So whether we bear children or not, we need to remember our power to mother all around us, including ourselves. When we embrace this mothering capacity—especially toward ourselves—we begin to untether from our dependence on others.

Through the embrace of our immense nurturing capacity, we take the mothering of our own self into our hands and end our psychological dependence on the external world. In this way, we elevate ourselves into the sacred realm of a goddess and feed ourselves with the worth we once thought could come only from the external world.

Reclamation of Ourselves

When there is a choice between whether the awakened woman should look outward or inward, she goes inward, and only then outward. By constantly checking herself before she commits to another, she reverses the effects of the original divorce in childhood where she severed from her truth. She declares to her loved ones that it is her greatest desire to be of service and that she is truly committed to the others' care, while at the same time clearly affirming her alignment with her inner voice. The others in her life, although reluctant to accept this at first, will eventually acquiesce, for they will see that she speaks from an inner knowing that isn't swayed by others, including threats.

Part of our awakening comes in the awareness and reclamation of our body and our sexual nature. Part of owning our body means getting in touch with our natural rhythms and cycles. Take our menstrual cycle. We are grossly out of touch with its peaks and valleys. In each of the phases of our cycle, our body goes through vast hormonal changes, many of which we are not in tune with. As a result, we work against our body's natural rhythm, and this asynchrony has a negative consequence on our psychology.

I never really paid attention to hormones' significant power over my psyche until I began to breastfeed. Now, as I approach menopause and speak to dozens of friends, I bow to the power of these internal chemicals. Our hormones uniquely set us up to carry the feminine principle. Every month, most of us are affected by the enormous power of our hormones as they trigger mood and appetite swings. The intricate manner in which our hormones interact with our biology profoundly influences our emotions on a daily basis.

Let's talk about the pill, shall we? When the birth control pill was invented in 1960, it marked a new way of being for women. In some ways, it liberated females and, in other ways, it ensnared them. It allowed women to have more sex with less risk of an unwanted pregnancy. It allowed females, married or not, to feel in greater control of their menstrual cycles and sexual expression. They could now plan out their fertility independent of their partners or spouse and give themselves opportunities to have careers for as long as they desired. Increasing numbers of women began to get college educations and earn more. The age of marriage was gradually pushed later and later. There was greater freedom of choice and, with this, an increased sexual expression.

But with all good things, there are downsides. So it is with the pill. The downside is that it takes us out of our body's natural rhythms and this comes with its own consequences. There is a price to pay for working against how nature intended. Many women complain of weight gain, bloating, severe PMS symptoms, irritability, and crankiness. This cannot be positive for us by any means. Part of awakening involves doing the research it takes to educate ourselves about our hormones and our choices. We need to make sure we are not simply driven to choices without empowering ourselves with knowledge.

As we begin to own our body and the choices we make, we are able to enter our sexuality in a more empowered way. Doing so allows us to break free from much of the sexual suppression the patriarchy has had over us. *Sex* is not a dirty word anymore and the experience isn't a shameful one in our minds any longer. Only when we undo the toxic conditioning we received do we end our dependence on men or others for sex. Part of this is learning how to orgasm and permitting ourselves to desire it as much as we want. This involves reimagining ourselves as sexual beings. Instead of hiding behind the veil of cultural dogma, we need to allow ourselves to flourish sexually.

When I began to own my sexuality, I found myself not only more connected to my body but also more accepting of it, which led to a reverence and celebration of it. This permitted a sexual transformation and blossoming, which I now own as an ever-evolving exploration, one which is now fully self-regulated by my autonomous desires and not by culture's dictates.

A woman who fully appreciates the immeasurable gifts and wealth her body holds is a formidable powerhouse. Once she fully gets in touch with exactly how amazing her body truly is, she goes beyond its form to its functional miracles. Beyond its physical beauty and its capacity for sexual pleasure, the fact that a woman's body can tend and nurture her young is a feat of unrivaled proportions. Once she understands the potential her body houses, and fully embraces what this means for herself, she can develop an intimate relationship with herself and her inner power. She now understands her strength and begins to harness its irrevocable energy. There is no holding her back anymore. She has found herself.

When this profound internal shift occurs, the highway is her magic carpet and her wheels are her wings. There is simply no stopping a woman who has reclaimed her own body. She now owns all she is without apology. She unabashedly occupies herself and isn't leaving anytime soon. All those around her have been served notice.

~

11

Two Different Biopsychologies

Clamoring for constant attention and care
The penis is wired for instant gratification and pleasure
It holds the man hostage to its vagrant needs
Leaving him bereft of free power over its demands
Trapped in his own private hell of pleasure and pain.

Most parents who have children of both sexes come into the shocking awareness of their acute differences. For the first time, perhaps, they are brought into the realization of how vastly distinct both sexes are. From their organic temperament, it's clear that boys and girls are constructed in unique ways. While some of this is cultural, there are innumerable biological differences that account for these psychological variations. Understanding these differences is key if we are to fully awaken to our sexuality with ourselves, one another and, through this, to our humanity.

It all begins with the male, whom nature holds responsible for its proliferation. It is he who holds the baton, so to speak. Nature gave males and females complementary roles, each playing a specific part in the reproductive dyad. Understanding what these roles are and how nature set them up gives us insight into how they have shaped our psychology and primed us for divisiveness due to culture's unconsciousness. Let's begin with how life starts with the ejaculation of the sperm through the male orgasm.

The first place to understanding just how different men and

women are in the sexual dyad is to wrap our brain around the fact that almost 100 percent of men reach orgasm every time during sex. While most women have the capacity to reach orgasm, a spectrum of studies has shown that only approximately 40 percent of women "nearly always" reach a climax during sex. Even here, these statistics are not consistent because they are influenced by many factors, such as whether the women are in loving relationships or feel connected to their partner.

I noticed this in my own sexual experiences. During sex, I was "searching" for that darn G-spot, craning my entire body, waiting for my orgasm, whereas my male sexual partners were trying desperately to *not* have one. This was a fascinating observation. Why was one trying so hard to climax, whereas the other was trying so hard *not* to? Was it just me, or was it almost always the case with women? This is when I did some research and was shocked at how universally challenging it was for the female body to reach climax.

The question this begets is, What's the significance of this difference?

Perhaps nature created this difference because the female's role in the reproductive dyad is different from the male's? The male is given the onus of proliferation with his millions of sperm. With this onus comes the guarantee of pleasure. He is aroused quickly and is able to orgasm speedily. If he wasn't guaranteed pleasure, he wouldn't readily carry out nature's imperative for him to procreate. His reward for carrying out nature's mandate to support her reproductive agenda? An intensely pleasurable orgasm.

Think about it: only one in the male–female dyad needs to orgasm and ejaculate in order for reproduction to occur. If nature gave both parties the need to orgasm in order to reproduce then, with it, she would give both the active role. She knew, though, that a healthy balance comes from a union of active and passive, of thrusting and receiving, of yin and yang. She bestowed the male with the active role and the female with the passive role, aware that both are pivotal in the dance of life.

With their more passive role in the dance, females don't need to have an orgasm to reproduce. They can become pregnant without it if copulation occurs within her fertility period. Nonhuman animals signal their fertility in all sorts of ways, from pheromones to vocal calls. Nature gave women protection against constant pregnancies by making her fertile during only a certain time of the month and, then again, only for a limited span of her life. If she is in her fertile period, she is likely to become pregnant if she receives a male's ejaculation. For a male? It's very different. He is always ready, but his orgasm is a must in order for reproduction to stand a chance.

Because he is guaranteed this pleasure, he is likely to seek it more than females. In this seeking, he will naturally call on his predatory instincts. Male predation exists in all of the animal kingdom. Yet there is little rape as we know it in the nonhuman animal kingdom, let alone other sexual perversions of the modern world. Culture has convoluted and perverted a natural way of being, resulting in a toxic masculinity that aggressively marauds its females without care for their vulnerability.

The Biology of the Male

The male penis is often referred to as his second brain. It is neurally networked in such a way that it can be aroused against the conscious volition of the man. I cannot tell you how many men have confessed to me in my sessions that they often feel embarrassed by the ease and frequency of their arousal because many times this is against their conscious will. Research has shown that the average man has about eleven erections a day, many of which occur at night, and often occur without any obvious sexual stimulation.

To ensure proliferation of the species, males need to be aroused easily and often. So how did nature set this up? She bestowed males with a greater sensitivity to visual stimulation than females. This difference is the reason many of us deride a male's "wandering eye." If we truly understood why their eye wanders, we would see that the vast majority of human males—i.e., men—cannot help themselves.

Let's stop a moment. Are you having a negative reaction to what you are reading? A reaction that calls "bullshit" on this? If you are, it is even more important for you to read this. I used to have this reaction too. I scorned and scowled at my male friends for turning their heads at every attractive female that passed by. I labeled them "immature" and even took it personally. It has only been of late, once I had done the research, that I entered a wiser discernment of these issues based on their biological roots. The reaction many women have is born out of the misconception that we are not animals. When we forget we are animals, we ignore how we are innately wired and, because of this, we suffer.

Men are wired to be aroused by visual stimulation. This is in their neurochemical blueprint. Failing to recognize this leads women to believe men are intentionally setting out to hurt them. This couldn't be further from the truth.

Entering a cinema one day, a friend shared with me that, momentarily, his eye was caught by a woman as she walked out of the cinema. He turned his head for just a second. Spotting what was happening, his wife screamed at him, "You lech!" Hoping to recover from this unexpected setback, he explained that he thought the woman was someone he knew. His wife didn't buy it and stormed out of the theater to catch a taxi home. There was no sex that night or for the next several nights.

Do you know how many men have complained to me about fights like this, where they might have gawked at a female form for too long and upset their wife or female partners? Where they are forced to lower their gaze and pretend they didn't notice an attractive woman, when actually all they wanted to do was stare? For them, it is akin to how we would feel gawking at a beautiful flower or a sunset.

What women don't understand, as I didn't for decades, is that the male response to the female form is *wired*. We think that when men turn their heads to look at an attractive female that it's an intentional choice and, therefore, take it as a personal slight. How wrong we are! It's all to do with biology. Nature needs her males to be on the move for her constantly and therefore gives him easy arousal so that he can do "his job." Women judge men without being curious about what it must be like for them to live under the constant siege of libidinal need.

A man's biological mandate is to sleep, eat, and have sex. Ours is, too, but the sex part is not as burdensome a mandate for us. Our ovulatory cycle lasts twenty-eight to thirty days, whereas men work on more of a twenty-four-hour hormonal cycle. This causes a man to feel sexual arousal far more often than many women. Sexual stimulation in a male is governed by testosterone and most men have about ten to fifty times more testosterone than women. This one hormone has the potential to create all the difference. The fact that testosterone courses through the male bloodstream at such a rate means they are under the siege of a completely different mindset than women.

Perhaps it is in how *oxytocin*—often known as the "cuddle hormone" or the "love hormone" because it is released when people snuggle together or bond socially—works differently in men and women that also contributes to women not being able to relate to how men handle their sexuality. For us, sexuality has a lot to do with connection. Perhaps most of what we do involves connection. Our oxytocin levels encourage us to prioritize connection and kinship. Our body's release of oxytocin during labor, for example, allows us to bond and tend to our child, something males don't experience. It's quite understandable that women don't understand how men can compartmentalize sex, apparently not needing the connection we so desperately crave.

I recognize that there is a complex interplay of hormones that need to be accounted for at all times. I am only touching upon these specific points in an abbreviated manner to draw attention to how inherently different men and women are.

Many a man has told me that searching for sexual relief is the same as foraging for food. What they mean by this is that, just like we feel the pangs of hunger on a consistent basis, they experience pangs for sex. This doesn't emerge out of a conscious choice but is more biological. It comes from the same impulse and has the same neutrality as looking for a restaurant to serve a particular cuisine. Do we deride our teens who seem to be hungry all the time? I see how I act when I am hungry for food. I am crabby, irritable, and childish. I literally want to tear my teeth into anything I can find. When I see how hunger affects me and I then correlate that same hunger with a man's sexual deprivation, I can understand how his hormones affect him.

With this understanding comes a deep compassion where I move away from blame, guilt, and shame into a new terrain of empathy. I fully own that as a woman I can only empathize but never fully know the reality of a man. More than this, I feel the urge to help them regulate their sexual hunger as opposed to shaming them. Just as a man can never know what it feels like to menstruate, be pregnant, undergo labor pains, give birth, or breastfeed, so women can never know what it means for a man to be captured by his sexual appetite and desire. Understanding this is key to liberating ourselves both within male-female relationships and our culture at large.

When a man constantly needs sex, women often get upset. We complain about their needs and refer to them as dogs or beasts. Sometimes our frustrations are justified. After all, we are on the receiving end of their predation, which can be downright exhausting. The fact is, many women shame men over their biological needs. We don't understand them, so we denigrate them. If we began to understand their needs, we would create a bridge toward them. Now, of course, there are some couples where the females have a higher sex drive than the males. This is not unusual. I am only speaking of the broad stereotypical experiences of most females and males around the world where the prevailing experience is that the males have a higher sex drive in comparison to females.

The awareness of how differently men are wired has the potential to bring forth empathy and compassion. Instead of seeing them as an enemy who is against us, we see them as struggling cohumans who need our understanding. We don't see their lust for sex with us or another as a personal affront to ourselves or our values but understand it within its biological context.

The hunger for sex is on a man's mind while the urge lasts, then it's out of his mind. In this manner, a man can manifest a certain degree of blunted affect around sex, along with an amazing capacity to compartmentalize. This leads them to sometimes objectify us in order to fulfill their almost-daily mandate to consummate their sexual pressure. Nature didn't mean this objectification to turn to abuse. Culture has done this through its brutal subjugation of women. Nature gave men a practical mandate, yes, but this doesn't equate to abuse. With this mandate, penetration of a female involved a functional quality. In, out, done. This is at least how it feels to us, so we scorn it even more. We judge men for being infantile in their need to have sex and simply move on.

We have vilified men for their high sex drive. Part of this is because we have felt prey to their unwanted advances. But another part of this is because we have not understood how nature set them up. Just like we shouldn't shame ourselves for finding our grandmother's recipe of lasagna or chocolate cake irresistible to the point that we yearn for it or overeat it when she makes it for the holidays, we cannot shame men for feeling this hunger for sex. Let's remember though in this high lust, nature didn't intend for the male to force himself on a female or dominate her violently. Patriarchy has done this.

Why do you think porn comprises the most viewed sites on the internet? Why is prostitution the oldest profession? Is it just because "men are pigs"? If we went with this explanation, wouldn't we be saying that our sons are future pigs? Does this sound right? Many women and some men will echo a resounding, "Yes! Men are pigs indeed." This would be their reaction because culture has done a great job at conditioning us to vilify male lust instead of understanding its science.

I am not advocating that men watch porn, visit strip clubs, or stare at buxom strangers. I am simply trying to understand *why* they are so drawn to do so on a biological level. It isn't enough for me to rest easy in judgment and shame. I want to dig deeper into how a man's innate wiring contributes to his sexuality. To understand this is to understand the way of the male *tao*.

By having a penis that he inserts into a vagina, a man is already acclimated to penetrating boundaries. Just by this act, there is some inherent violation of another, even if done in the most loving way. His thrusting requires aggression. By being outside of his body, the penis acts like a weapon of conquest. This is why, in part, males have an easier time being aggressive and dominating. When taken to an extreme, this manifests as toxic masculinity.

Our brothers and sons need help. They need to be educated about their bodies and their desires. Instead of feeling ashamed when they begin to feel horniness during adolescence, they need to feel celebrated and honored. They need to see their sexuality as divine, just as we see ours. When they do, they can be ushered into a consciousness that honors itself and its sexual partners as divine mirrors of nature herself. Such a consciousness cannot harm another. It can only elevate and exalt another. It all begins with a redefinition of sexuality and a rebirthing of a new sexual consciousness in men and women alike.

The Golden Egg

Sperm is cheap, whereas the egg is golden and precious. Men can ejaculate millions of sperm each time they orgasm. They produce billions each day. These numbers are staggering. It's the reason men are so cavalier about their seed. They can literally give it away and walk away without a care. Women, on the other hand? We ovulate one egg per month and we have a limited number of eggs per life cycle. They are with us when we are born and they start decreasing with each passing year. While a man is fertile through-out the month, a woman is fertile only when her one golden egg is released. This is how important her window of fertility is. Whom she gives that one egg to matters.

A woman's ovulation is not on display. Only she knows when her open window is. Nature protected us so that we would stay in charge of our fertility. We are meant to carefully select which mate gets our golden egg. Not everyone deserves the opportunity, only the one we deem most fit. That is why, in the natural world, males are the ones who pursue and seduce the females. The males need to compete for that one valuable opportunity to impregnate the golden egg.

When we understand this one fact—our different natural wiring—we begin to act very differently. Instead of trying to vie for the attention of men, we would expect *them* to vie for us. To-day, females are in constant competition with one another for the attention of men. How did things get so upside down? If we under-stood how nature intended it to be, we would stop our competition. Instead of contorting ourselves to seduce the males in our lives, we would do the reverse. We would know our worth and let them seduce us.

I see a plethora of young girls today caking their faces with makeup, wearing false lashes, Botoxing their cheeks and lips, taking out their ribs, implanting their bottoms, all in an effort to compete with other women. Why? To secure the attention of males. In this competition, we women hand our power to the patriarchy. Instead of owning who we are without apology and calling the men over to us, we do the opposite. We compete with one another mercilessly and manipulate ourselves into unnatu-ral shapes and disguises. We don't realize how this compromises our power and diminishes our worth. We think we look better on the outside. While this is subject to debate, what is more cer-tain is that we are denigrating ourselves on the inside and selling ourselves to the highest bidder, playing right into the patriarchy that we resent for controlling us. Do you see how we coparticipate in our own subjugation?

The tables need to be turned. We need to stop pretending we are the ones who lack. Men need us as much, if not more, than we need them. Why do we reduce ourselves to objects, then complain we are objectified? When we raise ourselves to the worth of the goddesses we truly are, we will demand and receive the respect we deserve. We need to realize that we may not be biologically endowed with physical power, but we hold within us what life needs the most to survive—our eggs.

Predator and Prey

By the time I was six or seven, I realized I needed to protect myself from men and told myself I needed to be a ninja warrior, even though I had zero clue how. By the time I was twelve, I had been molested by two males who were relatives, and had been mauled on buses, trains, and at family events by a few dozen male strangers. Possessing an eye color and skin tone that people in my country coveted, I received an undue amount of attention. As I grew and sprouted early breasts, I was a target for innumerable male advances. The amount of attention I received was more excessive than any young child should bear, and generated in me a wariness of men.

My mother was oblivious to what I was experiencing. She was clueless that I was an easy target and ready prey for young boys and men. How could she not see it? When I later shared with her what I went through, she was appalled. She had not experienced the extent of unwanted attention I received when she was growing up because she was protected by her strict parents. Sheltered by her parents, she herself grew up sexually suppressed. Unaware of male-female dynamics out in the real world, she didn't realize she needed to protect me against the predatorial instincts of the men who surrounded me.

When one particularly touchy-feely male relative would sometimes spend the night for some reason or the other, I would tie my blanket around my head and toes, sausage-like, pretending to be dead. It never worked. I was ballsy, though. One time, I actually shoved him off me, kicked him in his groin, and ran to my mom's room. When I later threatened to tell my mom, it still didn't stop him. He knew my nature—he had vetted me well. I was too softhearted to hurt my parents and deliver the psychological angst involved. Precocious and empathic, I decided I was strong enough to handle these inflictions myself rather than put them on my parents. I intuited that they would not be able to handle it. This meant this particular touchy-feely man won. I stayed silent. I soon grew resigned to his unwanted attention, followed by that of others.

The tragedy isn't just that these men did what they did to a defenseless young girl, as males do to millions of females around the globe. The real tragedy is that our mothers, aunts, and female teachers don't tell us how to prepare for it. No one told me that I was prey, but this is what I wish someone had explained to me. I wish someone had held me by the shoulders, looked deep into my eyes, and said, "You are a girl who will grow into a woman. From now on until old age, you will forever be preyed upon. Not all men see women as prey, but many do. Your awareness of this fact will be to your advantage. It will empower you. There is nothing to feel bad about—it's just the way of nature. By being aware of this, you won't be caught off guard. You will be vigilant, ever present. You will protect yourself as wisely as you can, knowing that even when you do so you will fall to unwanted advances. As soon as this happens, you are to call on your sisters or one of us. You are to reach out for help. You are to speak up and speak out against any abuse. There is no shame in being a victim of a predator. It is not your fault if this happens. Your smaller stature leaves you a ready prey for a man who hasn't tamed his instincts. But it doesn't make you victimized for life." Oh, how I wish someone had normalized what I went through, and that I felt free to express my confusion. The culture did not give me space to speak up, so I write these words now to empower mothers and daughters to go through similar experiences differently.

Am I endorsing the predator? Hardly. See, this is not even about the predator. This is about us, the prey. By understanding our status in this thing called life, we can actually liberate ourselves. Pretending things are otherwise is a mistake. I understand how this description of ourselves as prey may rankle you—however, being prey doesn't need to leave us victimized. Victimhood is a mindset. Being a victim of predators like I was when young is a real thing. It isn't conjured up or imagined. But having worked through my past, I no longer live in a victimized consciousness. As I have said before, there is a big difference between being a victim of a crime—as many of us are, and speaking up about it—and living in a victimized consciousness. We need to be aware of the difference.

Other animals don't protest if they are labeled *predator* or *prey*. These labels just refer to who is the hunter and who is the hunted. Nonhuman animals know where they are on the food chain and, in many ways, appear to accept this. They develop acute sensors and hunting skills based on this awareness. They protect their young and oversee their tribes with an enviable savvy, doing so because their instincts emerge from their awareness of who they are. Of course, some men have never preyed on women and would balk at the suggestion. The point is that males are *wired* to be the hunters. Their radar, whether acted upon or not, is always on the hunt for an attractive female.

Most women are sick and tired of being the prey. It's downright exhausting, frustrating, and, at times, enraging. As well as being humiliating, it makes us vulnerable. Whether we are directly approached or not, the fact is we are always silently being preyed upon. Let's take a moment to acknowledge just how aggravating it is for us women to constantly be on a man's sexual radar. The grocery store, the gym—*the gym!* The airplane, the mall, the club, the job. Everywhere we go, we are preyed upon. We feel eyes on us constantly, and at times we feel hands on us. Do men even know how it feels to constantly be preyed upon? Do they even have a clue?

The other day I was in an elevator with two of my friends when a young man walked in. He sauntered in the elevator where we already stood and didn't even look up from his phone. When he left the elevator, my friends and I marveled at his ease at being surrounded by three women. Each of us knew that had the tables been reversed and it was us entering an elevator with three men, we would have felt very differently. How many times have we had to walk a longer route because we were afraid of taking a shortcut through an alley? How many times are we relieved when we walk through a park at night and see women, not just men?

On some level, men know they are predators. They also know that no one is preying on them. What a huge relief and freedom that must be. I cannot even imagine a day in the life of such freedom. Women need to be constantly on the defense. This is our lot as women, and the sooner we accept this without victimhood, the better.

Despite knowing we are prey, we are still not fully aware of just *how* preyed upon we are. If we think there is one man eyeing us, be prepared for the reality that there are ten more, we are just not aware of them. If we understood this, we would empower ourselves by surrounding ourselves with our sisters in dangerous situations as much as possible. When something untoward happens to us, since we don't have ultimate control over who we encounter, we would speak up and get the help we need.

Many of us have mistaken the act of being preyed upon as caring. We think, "Aww, he is so enamored with me. He thinks I am beautiful, so he must be serious about me." Or we may tell ourselves, "I think he likes me because he bought me flowers." Little do we realize that this is all part of the hunt. He doesn't necessarily like us any more than he likes the next woman he will prey upon. In his eyes, women are not entirely unlike a line in a buffet and he is going down the line looking for what's ready to be served. I know I sound crass, but ask most men and they will admit this is true—the single men, that is. Married men would never commit hari-kari by being this honest.

So many times we fall under the illusion that a man's attention means he cares. When he pursues us, we believe he is really interested. Then when the man discards us after a sexual encounter, we bemoan the fact. Little do we realize that we were never truly cared for, just preyed upon. This is such a hard but vital fact to accept and teach our daughters, isn't it?

By not understanding the nature of the hunt, women fall for unavailable and straying men, or we get hurt when the man we love shows another attention. I cannot tell you how many women come to me complaining about the men they date. They cannot believe how men seem to move on after sleeping with them, even after being with them for a while. We don't understand it and take it personally. We cry our guts out, lose sleep, and turn ourselves into anxious wrecks. If only we understood male psychobiology, we wouldn't waste our time shedding useless tears. We would arm ourselves against being preyed upon as much as possible. We would discern more carefully whom we sleep with. We would ask the right questions and not be beguiled by roses and sweet words. We would understand the nature of the hunt and play our role intelligently.

Even if we give ourselves to the most worthy suitor, we should never do so without being conscious of what it truly means. As we evolve, this worthy suitor would be one who understands his own male psychobiology and owns it fully. Such a man will not use a woman without disclosure of his intentions.

The reason so many of us claim to be hoodwinked by the men in our lives is that we are naive. We allow men to sweet-talk us without realizing we are probably simply a means to an end. Is every last man on earth like this? No, but the majority are.

This is not meant to be an exposé on males but simply an invitation for women to understand what's happening to them when they feel rejected. For the most part, it has little to do with them personally and has everything to do with the nature of the predator-prey dynamic. When we understand this, we suffer less.

Understanding our male partners in terms of their biological wiring means to understand whom we are dealing with. It's not really a question of whether we like this or not but more of a question of understanding the reality of things. Understanding allows us to create empowered choices. Once we understand the males we share our planet with, the more we bolster ourselves with wisdom and occupy inner freedom.

The Wisdom of Our Differences

One of the fundamental problems I have observed in relationships emerges from the idea that men and women should be alike. As I learn more about our inherent makeup, I have come to realize that this idea is a fantasy. In fact, it's the illusion that we need to be alike that causes much of the suffering we see in male–female relationships.

When we enter a male–female intimate relationship, it's natural we are going to experience major differences between us. This is normal for any relationship, really, but more so in a male–female dyad. As I outlined earlier, our wiring is so vastly different that it's almost an illusion to think we could be on the same page. When we can't connect, our needs go unmet. We enter a state of dissatisfaction. Restless, we either go inward through depression, or outward, possibly through straying. This disconnection often causes us suffering. Much of it is unnecessary and would fade if we understood that our fundamental problem is not in trying to mate with the opposite sex, but the fantasy that we need to experience life in exactly the same way.

We are inherently dimorphic. That is, there are two distinct forms of our species—male and female. This is true of not only our physical and sexual differences but also our psychological, emotional, and spiritual differences. To put two humans so inherently different under one roof and cut them off from the larger lifeblood of community is, in many cases, a recipe for disaster.

Pair bonding between males and females in long-term monogamous nuclear units may be one of the fundamental causes for relational dysfunction, domestic violence, and divorce. When you put two highly dimorphic adults who are largely unconscious into a binding legal contract, ask them to stay undyingly loyal to each other no matter how at odds their libidos are, then ask them to raise children together no matter how different their parenting philosophies, you have a prescription for failure. This is why most marriages collapse and why most who remain often reduce themselves to business and social transactions only.

Does this mean couples can never get along? Not at all. I am speaking to the widespread dissatisfaction that exists among couples and I am not talking about any individual couple per se.

Couples who wish to transcend cultural barriers are those who are willing to open their relationship to new possibilities, both sexual and emotional. They are open to discussing how their sexual differences are impacting each other and how this leads to emotional closeness or separation. Such couples may be able to be more consciously intentional of each other's sexual and emotional needs, allowing a variety of sources that may go beyond the monogamous dyad to fulfill these needs without the jealousy or possessiveness that obstructs a traditional couple's harmony.

By moving away from community into nuclear isolation, we live farther from our tribe and put more pressure on our partners to fulfill all the needs that were originally meant to be met by others in the village. Until we recognize this misalignment and live within communal networks like all the other animals, we will feel disenfranchised and lonely.

Our pair bonding isn't supposed to be our be-all and end-all in terms of emotional connection and sexual sustenance. It's simply unsustainable to demand that one singular person meet all of our emotional and sexual needs. For some of these, we may sometimes need to draw on others from our community. This is a healthy outlet. We "outsource" these needs, not out of belligerent rebellion but out of a wise acceptance that our partner may not have the same drives we do. When we allow for our needs to be met through a variety of ways, we engage in our primary relationships with greater enthusiasm and wholeness. The best way to do this is through engaging in a larger community.

Kibbutzim, communes, and other intentional communities have long existed and continue to exist around the world. Such groups understand the pivotal importance of living on shared land with shared resources and relationships. Children are raised by a vast network of adults, allowing them to create their own web of interdependence. In this way, children can count on several adults to raise them and don't have to rely on the limitations of their biological fathers or mothers. For adults, as well, the tribe offers greater options for emotional and sexual outlets and fulfillment. When the community sets its intention on sacred sharing, adults are able to manage multiple relationships without encountering the ownership and control elements that plague a traditional dyad.

This is not to eulogize these kinds of communities as somehow utopic, but to recognize that all animals, including humans, have lived in these communal ways throughout history. The current nuclear monogamous dyad is a modern invention, one that has borne severe psychological, sexual, and emotional costs for both the individual and the family. Its penchant for disintegration and dysfunction is not due to a lack of morality or effort but due to its departure from our inherent nature as biological and communal beings.

Intentional spiritual communities have been one of the pivotal factors of transformation in my life. When I use the word *intentional*, I mean consciously created and deliberately intended. When we associate with our long-standing family and friends, there is often a sense of obligation and duty. There may also be a sense of a misaligned purpose, which doesn't exist in an intentional community. Here, people gather together out of a common vision and mission. They often speak a common language, one that the soul understands, and they come together for the purpose of inner transformation and connection—be it just emotional or with an additional sexual component.

How to find such an intentional community? The first thing to do is become clear about your intention from within. As you start aligning your own speech, behaviors, and actions, you branch outward. You begin joining groups that reflect this alignment. In my own life, I began to "hang out" in the communities of people whose wisdom I admired, and then created my own gathering spaces where people from all over the world could join in. Through these intentional connections, I gave myself permission to be authentically me. Partaking in such communities takes action. It isn't a passive process you can just wait for. One needs to pursue these connections. It is the move from passivity to activity that we, as awakening women, need to engage. As we do so, we move away from that which no longer serves us to that which does.

As we take these conscious steps, we begin to contour our lives to reflect all that we have felt within our soul and only now are courageous enough to manifest. Living among those who match our inner essence is not just a gift we give ourselves, but it is our right as awakening beings.

~

Part Four

CRACKING

the

MATRIX

~

12

Fact or Fiction?

In a haze of lies, we can't know truth
In a quagmire of shame, we can't know sovereignty
In a web of duplicity, we can't know authenticity
Much of what we have been conditioned to believe in is false
The quest for our essence begins in this discovery.

The lies culture tells us didn't begin with us. They seeped into the minds of our parents, as they did with their parents before them. Never having had the chance to wake up, our parents unwittingly believed these lies and raised us to believe them as well. What happened next was pivotal. We imbibed these voices *as our own.* Now those voices are our voices. *We cannot tell them apart from ourselves.*

We women have lost ourselves down a rabbit hole of beliefs that are mostly unnatural. Because it's our nature to accommodate and submit to our loved ones, we don't question them. We naively follow, shrouding ourselves with false beliefs.

When I began awakening, I could hardly believe it was possible to think differently. It was unfathomable to me that I had any volition where these voices were concerned. I felt fated to believe they were who I was. Only when I realized that these voices were lies was I able, slowly at first, to detach from them.

Our conditioning is as deep and pervasive as the ocean is to a fish. We don't even know we are being conditioned. We are deeply indoctrinated from our earliest days, so it's natural we think this is the way the world works. If our parents told us to pray to purple porcupines that hide in the sky, we would. If they told us that the world was shaped like a triangle, we would believe that too.

I used to love a game my daughter played when she was young. It was called Fact or Fiction. At school, they learned the pivotal difference between the two. Facts are easily verifiable. The sun is hot, the earth is round, the shoe is blue, the wall is yellow. Fact—clear, observable, real. Nature doesn't need beliefs to be real. Rain is rain and gravity is gravity. The earth rotates and revolves around the sun. The seasons change when they do. The ocean creates waves or is calm. The sun produces heat and light. There's no disputing these realities, and therefore nothing to believe in. No one asks another person, Do you believe that it's raining right now? Do you believe that the sun gives us light? Nature is just what it is. We don't create wars around it, nor sects nor groups.

It's so obviously and painfully clear that our beliefs are simply that—*beliefs*. They prevent us from seeing what's right in front of us. Fiction is everything but facts. It's subjective and personal. Fiction includes beliefs and wishes, faith and hope—castles in the air, stories we humans create and to which we cling.

As we awaken, we realize how little our thought processes are based on facts and how much they are based on fiction. Just by saying "I believe," we are in effect saying, "I'm talking about something fictitious." If it was based on fact, we wouldn't need to believe. It would be right before our eyes for everyone to observe, touch, feel, and see. There would be no debate.

The Buddha understood that beliefs are false ideals we cling to because our mind is too weak to grasp the reality of things as they are. People believe in all sorts of things. The Hindus believe in the monkey god and the elephant god. The Jews believe they are the "chosen people." Others believe in chanting various prayers, as if they were charms that could change their fortunes. Most people have a belief, a story about some aspect of life or death. It's on these beliefs that we construct the gods we choose to believe in and serve, and which become the basis of our daily reality.

The Buddha also said that life is *maya,* meaning an illusion—things are not as they seem. What he meant is that our unique conditioning, histories, and emotional legacies color our perceptions. Our unawareness of this makes us feel that what we believe is real, yet much of what we see is the way we have been conditioned to see it. We see things as our mindset tells us they are, not as they truly are.

Culture and, in particular, the patriarchy are deathly afraid of the awakened and empowered woman. She is a threat to the status quo. A woman who is no longer docile, quiet, servile, and dependent? No longer willing to compromise her worth for another's comfort and well-being? No longer willing to take second place except when she consciously chooses to do so?

That woman?

Do you know what power she houses within her? She is a force to reckon with. She is a woman who has tasted the nectar of her own endorsement. She is unstoppable. She cannot be shackled by fear anymore. None of the old ways work with her. She sees through the mirage of it all. When her life touches others, they feel this freedom in their own lives. Soon all are liberated to live in truth. Such a state of being can never harm another, for each one's essence is honored. A woman who honors her own essence has the power to truly heal the world.

To awaken means we stop playing to the tune of the outer world and instead start expressing ourselves according to our inner world. Once we understand that we have been living an *idea* of who we are versus the truth of who we are, we begin to peel away all that doesn't match our authentic self.

A Dysfunctional Lie

Most of us were raised on a strict diet of myths, beliefs, and illusions spun by our parents and our culture. Our parents, for the most part, were also pawns to the culture. As a result, their own minds were imbued with whatever beliefs-du-jour saturated their environment. Without thought to whether they were legitimate, logical, reasonable, conscious, or not, they simply ingested these beliefs as their own. They ended up in our milk bottle and baby food, spiced with ingredients that were as familiar as the air we breathe. No one sought to challenge or defy the status quo.

If culture says that drinking two-and-a-half quarts of milk and eating four eggs at breakfast daily is healthy, we robotically follow this advice. Or we eat chicken, or rats, or snails. What difference does it make at the end of the day? It's all conditioning, don't you see? In some countries they eat spider legs and crickets—not because they are strange but because this is how they were raised. To another culture, eating chickens may be weird. Once we understand that it's all a matter of programming, we see how most of the algorithms of our upbringing were manipulated by a culture that largely profited from its propaganda.

Take the simple example of Valentine's Day, where we have been herded into this idea of romance and courting. Roses, jewelry, candlelight dinners, cards, balloons, teddy bears, and chocolates have been sold as the trademark expressions of this occasion, giving women the false idea they are somehow only loved and coveted if their partners gift them with such expressions of romance. Men certainly have fallen into the trap as well, feeling pressure if they fail to provide their partners with all the bells and whistles of the holiday. As a result, huge bouquets of flowers arrive, sometimes coupled with lavish gifts professing love. We succumb to the belief that love needs to be celebrated this way without fully realizing we are pawns in a large, commercialized system making millions.

The same is true of the diamond industry, which has also hugely profited from the idea of romance and love. De Beers and the pioneers of the diamond boom were able to convert the perception of pebbles as the most prized jewels. This is just another example of how we have bought into systemic customs without realizing we are being played by consumerism.

Most of us are raised on the beliefs of the day. When we were young, our childlike guile and innocence had us believing any-thing our parents told us, ranging from Santa, to the tooth fairy, to lucky four-leaf clovers. We never imagined we were stepping into utter falsities that would entrap us and shape our psychology for decades to come.

It's important to teach our children what's real. We don't need to take the fun out of the tooth fairy or take Santa away from them, but they need to know what's real and what isn't. If you have seen *The Truman Show*, you know exactly what I'm talking about. It's about a man who lives in a simulated reality show and doesn't real-ize it until he is an adult. We are like Truman in our own *Truman Show* bubble.

Peeling Away the Cultural Facade

Later in life, some of us dare to admit, "Hey, this doesn't make any sense." The result is often a backlash, and is one reason most par-ents and teens clash. The teenage stage of life is when kids are com-ing out from under their parents' spell, and they realize for the first time that they have been sold a bag of tricks.

Growing up, we readily believed that everything we are told had been tried and tested. We didn't know that the systems in place were unconscious, fear-ridden, corrupt, and that much of what we saw in magazines and the news was a lie. We couldn't imagine that our leaders would manipulate us, or that the government we trusted could betray us. Most of all, we couldn't believe that our parents would fall for all this and force it down our throats.

When teens begin to speak up and defy their parents' authority or the cultural traditions in which they have been immersed, they are often given a severe reprimand and labeled "disrespectful." When I began to awaken at twenty-two, I realized that much of what I thought was real was only a conglomerate of my inherited parental and cultural beliefs. Who was *I* then? What did *I* believe in? Was I just a hapless product of my upbringing? Was anything believable? I began to question everything—and I do mean everything. The more I questioned, the more I realized how most everything we are taught about ourselves and reality is smoke and mirrors.

When something happens to us in life, instead of entering the experience as it is, our instinct is to create stories around it. For example, if we were on top of a mountain and saw an exquisite sunset, we would marvel at our luck and label this day a good one. Similarly, if we climbed that same mountain another day, and were attacked by a mountain lion, or got caught in a massive storm, we might label it the worst day of our lives. Depending on the story we create about the day, we might return to the mountain often or never go back. The reality is that both days were simply days.

So it is with our personal relationships. Depending on the issues we bring with us from childhood, we constantly project our past onto our present and create mental movies around it, inventing good guys and bad guys based on our projections. This doesn't mean there aren't enemies out there. All I am saying is that much of what we think we see is more about *how we think* than it is about actual reality.

Our lives are not really our lives but are based on our *beliefs* about our lives. Can you imagine how many opportunities we missed because of misguided beliefs? How many mountains we didn't climb, how many paths we didn't walk, how many people we failed to get to know? I have seen countless people in therapy who wrap their lives in beliefs that are entirely false and ward off life's adventures because their minds won't allow them to venture out of their cage.

What would it be like to be raised without beliefs? We don't need to believe in anything. We only believe because we are too afraid of knowing reality as it *is*. Reality is impermanent, a fact too hard for most humans to fathom. If life is impermanent, then the truth is that all our attempts at control are ultimately meaningless. At the end of the day, we are all going to die, and we haven't a clue how or when. Ah, this is why we create beliefs, giving ourselves a *raison d'être*. We create beliefs to fake a sense of control over the uncontrollable nature of life. Beliefs assuage our anxiety that we are actually nothing more than a mote or a grain of sand. For me, this is an invigorating fact that allows me to understand myself at a deeper level. For another, it might be an abysmal reality that must be avoided at all costs.

Life is filled with unknowns. We don't know why someone is born in one type of home with riches, while another is born diseased and destitute. The Hindus sometimes simplistically believe that these differences in our life come from the way we lived in previous lives. The problem with this approach is that there is a presumption of good or bad. In some circles, rich people are automatically considered good and the destitute are considered bad. This leads to bias and stereotyping. The truth is, we don't know why or how we were born into the circumstances we were. We just were.

The fear of not being in control over the grand design of life and death has us searching for control in all sorts of ways. One of the most pervasive ways we have done this is through the creation of institutions. These institutions have rules and norms we cling to that allow us to feel in control. Little do we realize, these are castles spun of air. We give them credence because without them we would feel utterly out of control.

Rather than enter the truth of the nature of reality, which is that it *is* out of our control, we create surrogate realities that allow us to feel as if we know. This is the grand heist, the great delusion. We believe we know things when, in fact, we don't.

Because beliefs vary between each individual or culture, our reality is subjective. Otherwise we would all endorse the same reality because it would be the only reality there is. The fact that everyone has their own take on reality is the clearest demonstration that all of it—*all* of it, without any exception—emerges from the subjective reality of a person and their culture.

When we can't see the truth and prefer to create distortions of reality, even when they defy science or objectivity, we are treading on dangerous ground. We celebrate our faith in our beliefs and consider them sacred. The more faith we have, the more sanctified we feel. It's only when we begin to examine our own mind and realize how much it has been contaminated by beliefs that we let go of our attachment and enter a space of inner liberation, lightness, and empowerment.

Separating from the Mainstream

Awakening enables us to realize that we have been prey within a system of greed. From the education system, the beauty industry, and the tech industry, we are sold products that calm our fears. In order to take charge of our life, we need to crack the code of the matrix and transcend the pressure to subscribe to it. Only then can we ever hope to be free of the herd mentality that grips most of us.

Releasing our beliefs feels terrifying because we wonder who we will be without them. We think they empower us, when in fact they limit us. We believe that we will be nothing without our beliefs, when in fact the opposite is true. We only realize who we are when we are stripped of them. Instead of finding that we are nothing, we find that *they* are nothing. Instead of finding that we need them to survive, we realize that they have blocked us from thriving.

The greater the number who subscribe to beliefs, the greater the chance it's fictitious. The masses like to conform. They are typically superficial, trite, and disconnected from their authentic voice. If you are part of a mass group, you may find yourself willing to forgo your inner voice to be part of the crowd. The moment you begin to sing your own tune, you stand out.

Being part of the masses is not the same as being part of an intentional tribe or community. The masses are filled with followers, not unique thinkers. An intentional tribe, gathering, or community is the opposite. It seeks leaders and challenges each person to walk their own path, albeit within the sacred container of the larger network.

When we awaken, we choose to live by fact more than fiction. I often refer to this as living according to the as-is and not the as-if. We step out of denial and confront our life in a direct and transparent way. We refuse to silence our truth because it makes others uncomfortable. Our connection to ourselves is too vital and powerful to dismiss anymore.

The ultimate quest is to commune with reality as it appears before our eyes, without distorting it to fit a story. The more we become one with the is-ness of our world, the more we enter the present moment. The more we live in the present moment, the less we suffer. It all starts with our willingness to take our blinders off and begin communing with the reality of our lives instead of with fantasies. It takes a lot of daring to see through the webs of the matrix we live in, yet it is only by doing so that we can wipe them away and begin to see our world with clear vision. Until then, we will be colored by culture's deceits and maintain perceptions that are filled with delusion.

When we see how we have been fed a diet of false belief systems and have lived a life of unconscious unworthiness, we begin to take our power back. Once we claim our worth, we give ourselves permission to walk away from all that no longer serves us. We stop dancing to the fiddle of the other's view of us and take our approval back into our own hands. There will no longer need to be anyone on the outside to validate or deem us worthy. We will be enough in ourselves.

That is the kind of woman each of us has the potential to be.

13

The Lies About Love

So many ills in the name of love
Ownership, betrayal, control, need
So many shoulds, if-buts, when-thens said with a tongue of love
This is not true love. These are falsities in the name of love
These are lies that blaspheme the true nature of love.

Although love isn't an institution, per se, our modern-day idea of it has kept women locked in its cages. When we understand why this idea of modern love is more enslaving than it is liberating, we will revise what it means to truly love another and thereby free ourselves from the pain relationships often endure.

Most of us in the modern era were raised with fairy-tale notions of finding that one magical soulmate with whom we could live happily ever after. We were told that two halves make a whole and there is someone out there designed precisely for us who is the missing piece to our puzzle. Until we find this special someone, we are incomplete and, therefore, lesser than what we could otherwise be.

Sold on this idea of a "forever love" with another, diamonds are collected as the trademark symbol of the man's commitment toward the woman. Millions of romance novels and movies revolve around the idea that falling in love is a pivotal life experience worthy of ballads, poetry, and musicals.

Little girls and their mothers especially dream of a lavish wedding, which they look forward to with bated breath and eager hearts. Every boy the girl dates after the age of twenty-three is seen as a prospective husband. As they grow past the age of twenty-five, the need to hone in on the perfect mate becomes urgent.

Marrying the right person implies living "happily ever after." There is a definite agenda to all of this "falling in love." Love in this fashion is extremely goal driven. One doesn't love for the sake of loving. One loves for the sake of committing one's future to the other. One doesn't love as an expression of the soul, one loves as an expression of the ego's desire to fulfill an agenda.

Ask yourself, have you ever loved just for the sake of loving, or was your love always tainted with a future goal? If you are truly honest with yourself and look back on your past relationships, you might admit that within weeks or months of meeting your current partner, you looked at him or her in terms of marriage material.

The pattern goes something like this. Girl likes boy or girl, they date, and girl looks for a commitment of some sort, such as a ring signifying marriage. If the partner doesn't "commit"—a.k.a., ask the girl to marry him—the partner is considered to be not sufficiently loving. The market belief is that if the couple truly loves each other, they would marry because it's through the act of marriage that they declare their ultimate commitment.

What begins as a pure feeling from the heart quickly turns into a transaction for the future. We have been conditioned to be in a state of lack and scarcity. If we don't find someone to complete us, we fall into the trap of unnecessary suffering when a relationship doesn't reach the fruition of commitment. This sort of agenda takes our love, which is ephemeral and formless, and stuffs it in a box that is not only rigid but also future-based. We are thereby transplanted from the present, which is a felt experience of the moment, to the future, where we are trying to control the unknown.

The cultural script tells us to *fall in love with someone who completes us*. Besides the obvious implication that we are not whole enough without the other, the other more insidious undertone is that we are dependent on that person for our identity. The one we love is not just the receiver of our love but also part of the plan to gain a new identity as a whole person.

The implications of these beliefs are many. Let me explain through the example of a couple named Amy and Jacob. Amy is a classic empath. She came for therapy complaining about her relationship with her longtime partner, Jacob. She incessantly complained about his self-absorbed, narcissistic ways. It was easy to support Team Amy and cast Jacob as the enemy, since he clearly had no compunction about violating her boundaries and being insensitive to her needs. I realized, however, that if I supported Team Amy, I wouldn't help her develop into the whole person she needed to become. The goal was for Amy to understand what psychological function she was asking Jacob to fulfill for her, and how her own incomplete self was perpetuating this dynamic.

"What do you wish Jacob to be that he isn't being?" I asked.

"Patient, complimentary, loving, kind," she responded.

I asked her to complete the sentence "like who . . . ?"

She immediately said, "A father should be with his daughter."

The reason Amy was unable to see Jacob for who he truly was was that she was looking for a loving father to take care of her. As long as she had this need, she would stay dependent on a fantasy of who her partner should be but could never become.

"How do you act around Jacob?" I inquired.

"Scared, afraid to speak up, avoidant," she admitted. I asked her if this is who she used to be around her actual father and other authority figures. "A hundred percent," she agreed. "I was always the good, obedient girl who wanted to please everyone."

Amy was still trying to get the approval of her father and was bending over backward to do so. The pivotal difference she couldn't appreciate was that Jacob *wasn't* her father. Because she still had this need within her, she was walking around like a scared little girl looking for daddy's approval. Thus she cast Jacob in the role of her authoritarian father.

Jacob, on his part, is a man who tends to be self-absorbed and self-centered, probably exactly like her father. Left to themselves, there is nothing wrong with these traits. However, in a relationship, these traits are problematic because Jacob tends to violate the other person's boundaries in order to get his needs met. When one is in a relationship with a partner such as Jacob, strong boundaries and a sense of self are a requisite. If boundaries are not clearly established, the boundary violator will increase their behavioral patterns even more.

Amy grew up with a father who never recognized her boundaries. As a young girl she adapted by capitulating to him, craving his affection and attention. All she knew how to do was relinquish her boundaries. She developed into the perfect pleaser, using this persona to gain approval. As a result, she typically found herself taken advantage of and frequently abused. Jacob was one more in a long line of such people she had found herself intimate with.

Although she thought she was falling in love with Jacob, she was actually falling into an old pattern. She didn't recognize who Jacob truly was because her own unmet needs caused her to wear blinders. As she was looking for "daddy," she kept playing the role of "the little helpless pleaser." It could be said that she was in her own movie. Had she come to the relationship complete in herself, she would have recognized Jacob's tendencies and either never dated him in the first place or, if she chose to, proceeded to create healthy boundaries.

Amy is not alone. For most of us, this "falling in love" feeling is actually a falling into need, possession, control, and familiarity. It's a desire to fulfill something within ourselves. We believe we love the other but, in truth, are seeking love for our own ego. We fantasize that we are two grown-ups who are going to walk off into the sunset happily ever after without realizing that we are operating like little children instead of adults. We want the other to finish the work we haven't yet done to complete our own upbringing. We are adults who are emotional toddlers. Despite our tuxedos and ball gowns, we are ill-equipped to party with the grown-ups.

When we don't fully grow up, we constantly project our needs onto others and leak our emotions all over them. We want them to be the person we need to complete our fantasy of ourselves. The greater the childhood loss, the greater the fantasy and, thus, the greater our need for others to fulfill the role of savior.

I call this dynamic "twin beggars," each looking to the other to fill them up, their arms outstretched toward the other, hungry for the other to give them the magic potion they have been missing all their lives. What they don't realize is that they are each as empty as the other.

Because both people are dependent on the other, the desire to control and possess the other is palpable. They create unspoken conditions where expectations run high and the demand on the other is great. This naturally leads to control and possession. If we see the other as responsible for completing us, it's natural we will want to control the other. On this path, love morphs into its opposite. Instead of being about liberation and empowerment, it majors in possession.

When our sense of identity depends on another, we forsake our individuality in favor of the relationship. When two halves try to become one, they actually become quartered slivers of themselves. Lack always begets more lack. Only bounty creates bounty. This is why our modern-day understanding of love must be transformed. Before we can love another, *we absolutely must first learn to love ourselves irrevocably and meet our own needs.*

Most of us don't love—*we need, depend, possess, and control.* To put this differently, most of us don't love—*we fear.* Imagine the heartbreak when the other we have depended on refuses to bend to our fantasies and turns out to be who they truly are in their ego self, not the balm or salve we thought they would be.

When we enter a relationship with the intention of healing ourselves, conflicts or betrayals are no longer perceived as contentious but, instead, as powerful portals for inner integration. When we commit to looking in the mirror, we see our reflection everywhere. The more we heal and love ourselves, the more the reflection of the broken little child fades and gives way to a powerful and whole adult.

The Nature of True Love

Love is a powerful feeling toward another. Complex, nuanced, and multilayered, it is chemical, physical, emotional, psychological, and spiritual. It exists on the level of energy, undeniably passionate, and yet ephemeral and essentially unquantifiable. It's a force that can only be felt but never really be made solid.

To love someone is to feel for them without our own feelings about ourselves getting in the way. This is extremely hard to do for someone who hasn't worked on meeting their own needs, and therefore I call it "high" love. This shift from self to other is the mark of the higher nature of authentic love.

Poets and mystics have tried to describe such love for centuries, but all have fallen short of capturing its true nature. The reason is that love exists beyond the limits and boundaries of the form-based world. It doesn't exist for just one type of person or within the bounds of time, place, race, or creed. One doesn't just love dark-haired people who have short hair. Nor does one love only between the hours of 8 a.m. to 11:30 a.m. on Wednesdays.

At its core, love is a "free" emotion. What this means is that it is impromptu, unpredictable, accidental, and unintended. It occurs naturally and spontaneously. It cannot be forced, suppressed, planned, or organized. It cannot be contained. Because it's alive, it constantly changes, as do all living things. It simply doesn't stay the same but evolves. To bottle it up in a formula is to kill its essence and void its true spirit. To tell it how to express itself, when and with whom or for how long, is to suck the beauty of love's essential nature and convert it to another feeling—maybe still a worthy feeling but not the one we associate with love.

Because true love exists beyond the mind and the duality of "you and me," it can only be experienced in its transcendent state by those who recognize that love doesn't emerge from checklists or deadlines. It has nothing to do with logic, reason, or will. It's something that spontaneously combusts. While we need to use discernment, for sure, the feeling of love cannot be turned on or off like a switch.

Those who experience this kind of love often use exalted adjectives to describe it, such as *big, high, deep, transcendent, otherworldly*, and *spiritual*. Simply calling it *love* feels limited, because this kind of love *is* limitless, existing beyond self or other. Those who have been touched by this kind of love feel as if they have experienced the mystical magic of the heavens. They understand that they are living in the rarefied air of the privileged.

Love is the ultimate energy. It is *the self fully actualized*.

Not everyone is ready to experience this kind of love. It's reserved for those who have done the work of releasing their ego such that they are able to enter a space where they live unbound and untethered. It's only when the self has left its own self-absorption behind that this kind of love can enter one's consciousness.

This kind of "high" love doesn't ask to be returned or matched. It just loves for its own sake. It gives for free. Because its essential nature is freedom, it needs to be allowed to happen freely and needs to be released freely. It has no obligation or duty. It is wild and untamed. It just is what it is—authentic, honest, transparent, and raw. No frills, no adornments, no embellishments, and free of laws, loopholes, binders, promises, or conditions.

As long as we see love as an achievement of our identity, we will forever be enslaved by its presence in our life and never truly be free of its shadow emotions: hate, betrayal, rejection, or abandonment. These shadow emotions stem from a faulty notion of love.

As the parent of a girl rapidly moving toward adulthood, I am aware of the traps culture is laying out for this developing young woman. I try to combat them by teaching her there is no one to love on the outside and that the only person she needs to fall in love with and marry is herself. I remind her that culture sells us stories that are mostly false and she must never fall to the pressure of following the crowd.

No matter how hard I try, I cannot counteract all the images she imbibes from social media and her peer group. She watches celebrities on reality TV vying to fall in love with that perfect other, and sees the media hyping wedding days. Even though my voice is only one in the din of many, at least she is aware there is a different possibility for herself. This is where my power lies. I may not be able to change culture for my daughter, but I can certainly express an alternate path through my voice and the ways in which I carry myself in the world.

Self-love and growth should be the main criteria upon which we base our decision to be intimate with another. The prerequisite checklist of dating questions should be:

Do you love yourself? How do you express this?
How do you prioritize self-help and self-growth?
How do you honor who you authentically are?

These should be the questions we ask on a date instead of what jobs the other has held or what hobbies they have. If we truly want to test how loving another person will be, we need to measure the time they spend on loving themselves from within and the amount of energy they put into their growth.

Healing brings freedom from within. This, in turn, manifests as freedom on the external level. When one is free from within, one will become the greatest shepherd of another's freedom. Only those who violate their own inner truth violate the truth of others.

The Shift to Transcendence

Returning to Amy, she was stuck playing the role of a sweet, pleasing little girl trying to get her "dad," a.k.a. her partner, to approve of her. When the person she had cast in this role couldn't fulfill the function, she felt disappointed and hurt. Because she was trapped, she was unable to treat Jacob the way he needed, with clear and strong boundaries, which would perhaps correct his course and help him grow. Stuck in her own movie script, Amy did passive-aggressive things like complain, whine, and feel helpless and victimized, none of which helped Jacob stop violating her boundaries. On the contrary, this further emboldened him to continue with his abusive behavior.

When I told Amy she needed to focus on her own undeveloped self and not Jacob's behavior, she protested. She thought that meant I endorsed him or didn't fully validate her experiences. It's hard for us to be accountable for ourselves, isn't it? Little do we realize that feeling victimized by another is a source of energy depletion, not empowerment. By blaming another, we feel powerful but only momentarily. When stuck in a childlike version of ourselves, being seen as the "good one" is an important goal. If only we realized how stuck this keeps us. Wanting to be perceived as the good one is a craving of the ego.

The true self doesn't need to be perceived by others or the self in any particular way. It just simply is what it is, authentic and free. When we awaken, we stop living according to a childish relic of ourselves and instead begin to live in accordance with the truth of who we are as adults. Instead of living within an infantile movie, we live more in alignment with our context as it is, and not as we wished it to be as children.

We move away from the *as-if* to the *as-is*.

Amy was living in her own deeply personalized movie written in her past, *as-if* it was repeating itself. It was only when she woke up to the realization that she was repeating old patterns that she began to live in the *as-is* and related to Jacob as he truly was, rather than who she wished he was. As she shifted within herself, she shed her little girl role and began to create strong and clear boundaries.

Jacob, in turn, was forced to shed his roles as well. He was forced to go through his own process of growing up and dealing with his own inner emptiness rather than parasitically using his partner for this function. Instead of depending on the other to parent them, each began to stand in their own adult power. This process of reparenting is crucial if we are to awaken. We will visit this concept more fully in a later chapter.

As the authentic self grows, the climate for inauthenticity changes and the tolerance for false roles and dynamics dissipates. What takes its place is a clear and intentional call for an authentic alignment of two souls who wish to know each other at the deepest level of wholeness.

When two whole souls unite, the unity they enjoy is neither contractual nor obligatory. The love they share comes from completion, not incompletion, and thus is devoid of need and a desire to control. The other is relinquished from any and all enmeshment. In this manner, they become free to be how they wish to be on the continuum of consciousness. Here, when each works on their own inner wholeness, the prize of each one's authenticity and freedom is preserved by the other. These matter more to the couple than meeting each other's needs. By releasing our dependency on another, we begin to live in a sovereign and autonomous way and are able to grow up. Love untethers itself from an unhealthy attachment and moves into the space of transcendence and liberation.

Because we are not used to seeing ourselves in such a light, at first this level of "grown-upness" seems strange. We have been so conditioned to be enmeshed, needy, controlling, and dependent that this level of autonomy feels downright weird. We were raised by our parents to be sheep, using their feelings as our feelings, their goals as our goals, their thoughts as our thoughts. We never learned to know ourselves as whole and divine beings in our own right. Instead of developing our own authentic self so that we were validated and loved by ourselves, we were taught to don masks and false roles in order to feel validated. Our parents thought we were part of *their* micro-worlds instead of part of the larger cosmos itself.

To truly love another means to truly love ourselves. To truly love ourselves means to know ourselves. As we awaken, we realize we have never truly loved our self fully because *we haven't even known ourselves*. To know ourselves means to go on a path of self-discovery.

This is what this book is awakening in you. As you embark on this path, you shed the false idea you had of yourself and enter a true alignment with your inner being. You begin to see all parts of yourself through the eyes of love and compassion. You accept yourself unconditionally. In this unconditional acceptance of yourself, you are able to do the same toward others as well. The separation between you and others fades. You soon realize it was an illusion after all. You realize that there is no such thing as rejection by another, only by yourself. You now begin to love yourself fully. You are now free to be yourself. This is the greatest love affair of all, the one with your true self.

This love doesn't need another in a dependent way. Because it doesn't need another, it doesn't seek to control or possess another. As this love emerges from a self that is bathed in inner wholeness, it doesn't suck on others for fulfillment. It moves from dependence to interdependence, from a linear relationship to a circular, mutually reciprocal one. It discerns where others are on the continuum of consciousness and allows them to be where they are. It honors the process others need to undertake in order to find their true self, even if this means they walk away. It lives in freedom and bequeaths this precious treasure to others.

This may appear to be a radical perspective on love but, in truth, it's exactly what conscious love is intended to be—unconditional, nontransactional, devoid of control and possession, empty of need and dependency.

Conscious love is transcendent love. What this means is that it touches a space beyond the "I" or "you" and enters a new space, one that is as vast and limitless as the sky itself. It has no boundaries and/or restrictions. It is eternal, free, and boundless. It is liberation incarnate.

~

14

The Lies About
Marriage and Divorce

Love's essence is sovereign and unhampered.
Indiscriminate and wild.
It is timeless and boundless. It knows no borders.
Yet church and law have dimmed its power and stolen its freedom
Restricted to only one person and caged in permanence
All else is considered treason, betrayal, and deceit.

When we prescribe marriage as the end goal of a loving alliance between two people, we institutionalize it. For many couples, marriage is "love in a prescription bottle." It's akin to taking the beautiful scent from a flower and bottling it as a perfume. While still possibly lovely, the perfume can never fully capture the original essence of the flower. So it is with the institution of marriage. I am referring to the institutional nature of the tradition, as opposed to how it looks for any individual couple.

This is not a case for or against marriage but simply an exposé of the reality of marriage *as an institution*. Of course there are happy marriages and even ecstatic ones. The aim is to teach our sons and daughters about marriage as an institution and allow them to make a personal decision about whether to participate in it or not—a choice many of us never imagined we were free to make.

When marriage was transformed from being purely a social contract between families for the sole purpose of keeping property under control to being a divine contract ordained under the auspices of the church, everything changed. Once religion got its claws into the marital contract, it branded its dissolution a matter of sin. By psychologically brainwashing us to stay within its confines unless we wished to "burn in hell," the marital contract became something sacred. The more we honored it, the more points we would score in heaven. If we dared to desecrate it, we were sure never to gain entry into the pearly gates.

In taking the uncapturable essence of love and bottling it as a requirement for a happy life, marriage not only dilutes the feeling of love much of the time but contaminates it with all sorts of artificial ingredients. It imposes boundaries and strictures, attempting to preserve itself through will, law, and, at times, force. These are diametrically opposed to volition, freedom, and a spirit of celebration.

The judicial system legalized and legislated our relationships, transforming love into something contractual, conditional, and prescriptive. Marriage thus turns love, which is essentially formless, into an agreement with a promissory note for all future moments. This is where many marriages turn stagnant, sour, and end in a stalemate. The spirit has long gone. Imagine if culture transformed its understanding of marriage and divorce and turned the existing archaic paradigm on its head. We would revolutionize how we love, relate to one another, and parent. We would move away from the current prescriptions around possession and control, opening ourselves to a more liberated and unconditional way of loving each other. Our relationships would stay fresh, sexy, and free. There would no longer be the bitterness of divorce.

In a conscious relationship, the connection between the couple trumps their social or religious standing. In such a relationship, the couple transcends the traditional definitions of marriage and finds meaning solely in the bond they share with each other. The ego of their individual selves is overshadowed by the essence of their relationship. They are able to truly manifest the highest meaning of love without the usual egoic manipulations of shame, blame, guilt, and regret. In this way, the marital vows of unconditional love come to life.

Marriage Out of Control

All forms of love are to be celebrated. Yet in modern culture, typically only those forms of love that end in marriage are deemed worthy. Marriage as an institution controls whom we love and how we show that love. It tells us that we are only to love one person for the rest of our life. Not only this, we are forbidden from expressing intimate affection of any kind with anyone but our spouse. If this is not suppressive of who we are, I don't know what is.

The institution of marriage has even sanctioned which gender, races, religions, and creeds get married, prohibiting all these possibilities at various points in history. Dictating whom we choose to enter unions with is to ransack us of our rights to exercise our free will.

The marriage contract says no one should ever be close to another outside the marital dyad. If one dares to venture outside, the contract could be considered null and void. The marital structure ramps up the personal ego of the two parties and exaggerates the feeling of separation and betrayal. All the beautiful love that the two thought they had for each other is thrown out the window.

The real culprit is the institution itself. In its attempt to be a long-lasting pillar of society, it petrifies the ephemeral nature of love and rigidifies it. In this manner, the institution of marriage fossilizes the living and breathing vitality that is the mark of love. By taking the beauty of love and converting it into all the things love isn't, marriage brings out pride, control, possession, and dominance.

When we understand that love is something that constantly shifts, morphs, and transmutes, we cease to control it. We understand its present-moment nature and allow ourselves to flow through troughs and fly over peaks without clinging to it. When we try to hold on to love beyond its expiration date, it becomes stagnant and is accompanied with bitterness, resentment, regret, and anger. If we understood that love is a living, breathing phenomenon, we would realize that binding ourselves to a long-lasting legal contract is to work against the authentic truth of love's nature.

Marriage is applauded for one thing above all—its longevity. There are specific gifts assigned to mark each anniversary of marital time. Paper, cotton, leather, fruits, or flowers for the first four years. Wood describes the fifth anniversary, tin the tenth. As one completes their twenty-fifth, fiftieth, sixtieth, and more years of marriage, then come the real gems, metals, and stones ascribed to these markers of time—silver, gold, and diamond, respectively. Until then, the achievement isn't really noteworthy. The quality of those years doesn't really matter. Nor does the degree of growth. We don't talk about marriage in terms of inner transformation. All we care about is the length of time two people spend together.

So brainwashed are we by the longevity model that we look at it in terms of "putting in the time," no matter how we feel while doing it. We have so bought into culture's idea of marriage that we are downright terrified to approach marriage in any creative way.

It's no surprise that divorce is considered a fate akin to death and not worthy of celebration. Considered a bad word by many, some are even unable to say the word, preferring to call it the "D" word. Many are terrified of terminating their marital contracts. Ask any divorced person about their shame in exposing their marital status and they will share how society frowns on them. It's as if the person is infected. Divorce is failure—avoid it like the plague. Happy people stay together "till death do them part."

Divorce is seen as an insult to the family ancestry and an attack on the culture's morals. Sacrifice and compromise, even when the two individuals are dreadfully unhappy, is often preferred over the cost of social ostracism. Many millions stay in marriages that are at least dormant and, in many cases, extinct.

The paradigm of marriage needs to shift away from longevity

into growth. When we make this shift, we no longer count success in terms of years passed but in terms of self-growth and lessons learned. When the longevity model transforms into the growth model, marriage will soar to the realm in which it needs to exist—that of true kinship, connection, and freedom.

When we recast the paradigm of divorce in terms of a stagnation of growth, we see it as more than just the end of a marital contract. Divorce, consciously defined, is now seen as a passage between the old and the new. While it may signify the end of a marital contract with our ex, it also signifies the beginning of a marital contract with ourselves.

Divorce is not against our ex at all. The true divorce is against our own fears and inauthentic self. It signifies the end of the falsities we were living with and the beginning of an era of authentic, honest, and transparent living. The divorce marks the end of all that kept us bound by convention. In its aftermath lies the potential for a renewed commitment to our truth and our freedom.

Beyond the Institution of Marriage

What did people do before the agricultural revolution? It seems like they lived in small packs of thirty to fifty people and set up nomadic communities in which men and women loosely paired with each other. The children were taken care of by the entire community.

When the plough was invented, food began to be grown in blocks of land, which tied people to the land in a way they hadn't been at any time before in our history as a species. We settled down, living in smaller units. When marriage was introduced, it was different from what it is today. It was mostly for practical purposes. In fact, it still is in most parts of the world. Families come together to keep or expand property interests. For centuries, it was the way men controlled their assets, namely their land, wife, and children. Marriage was created to keep units together, with the mother close to her children and the father responsible for their upkeep. It was also an easy way to ensure that the property stayed within the family and that the man was not raising another person's child.

Marriage was, and still is, heavily patriarchal. Ordained by men, often under the eyes of God and governed by the law, it's largely controlled by clergy, fathers, husbands, and/or male authorities. The place of the woman and her children is second to, and lower than, the male in the household. As such, while marriage might protect the woman from other male predators, it frequently doesn't protect her within the bounds of the marriage itself. Marital rape was legal in many US states right up until the 1970s.

Take the most common scenario. A girl just out of college walks down the aisle with a boy she's been dating off and on through college or high school. They take the marital vow to "love and care till death do them part." If they haven't already, they move in together. This is done by thousands every single day as we attempt to re-create the households we grew up in or dreamed of growing up in. I call it an adult version of "playing house."

It isn't our fault that this is the only model we know, but we need to become aware that it is just that—a model. It isn't a prescription served up by God and neither is it the only way to live. It's just a way of being that has evolved, perpetuated by a culture that follows traditions out of compliance. In this model, we pledge our allegiance to another for the rest of our lives, making a promise to love them forever.

I can hear many of you protesting that if there wasn't an underlying contract of loyalty and longevity, most marriages would "fall apart." If that happened, then our children would be at risk. However, some 60 percent of marriages are already "falling apart" in the United States. This demonstrates the fragility of the marital institution. Think about it: would you get on an airplane that had a 60 percent chance of crashing? You certainly would not. Yet millions keep getting married day in and day out. The reason? Cultural indoctrination.

If it takes a legal contract to keep two people together, the question one should ask is whether the two people should be together in the first place. Are we so numb to the idea of autonomy that we think loyalty and longevity should trump individual growth and liberation? This is really a clash between the old paradigm of loving and marrying and a new, bolder paradigm of loving and liberating. The fact is this: whether they have a contract or not, people change their minds. What sense does it make for a twenty-four-year-old, for example, to bear the cost of her decisions for the rest of her life?

The old way is to marry for the sake of companionship over time. Here longevity matters, regardless of the quality. The old way is to see marriage as the only way to raise children securely. The old way is based on fear, possession, and control. It operates out of lack and unworthiness. It's clearly time for a paradigm shift. If it weren't, more than 50 percent of marriages wouldn't end acrimoniously in divorce.

We need to shift into a drastically new model of marriage, one that is based on growth, not longevity. One where choice, abundance, and freedom are the foundational elements of the union, instead of fear-based obligatory and contractual bonds. If marriages were predicated on different ideals such as growth, respect, authenticity, and freedom, we would be living in a different world. In this new model, we would allow each other to grow and evolve without any impingement. We would understand if the other needed to move on to another person or to another phase of their life. We would release the other with equanimity. We would work things out amicably. We wouldn't need divorce courts or lawyers. We would leave behind lack and truly embrace abundance.

It takes daring and courage to topple an entrenched institution such as marriage. It takes a new and bold vision for ourselves and our partners, one where respect for the other's unique expression of self takes precedence over our own ideas of how things should be. When this happens, there will only be interconnection and mutual reciprocity. When the marriage comes to a close, the couple can celebrate this transition instead of feeling ashamed and ostracized. The entire institution of divorce would come tumbling down. Now, wouldn't that be a marvelous thing indeed?

Finding Courage Despite Stigma

Culture fosters a huge stigma against divorce, in many cases even when abuse is involved, with the woman often being told by those she is close to that she shouldn't overreact by leaving the marriage. In fact, there are even mothers who encourage other women to accept their situations as they are, encouraging them to stay for the kids or for the sake of social inclusion, even if there is maltreatment or abuse. They might say something like:

> Your kids will suffer, so it is better to stick it out.
> Well, he didn't break your nose.
> At least he isn't a drug addict.
> He provides for you so well, so ignore the other stuff.

Such suppression of our truth creates an inner split and we stop trusting ourselves. Abandoning our inner knowing is the real trauma. We begin to second-guess our inner wisdom and doubt our judgment.

We all know how we can sense when something is wrong, but culture has us making all sorts of distorted excuses for our reality. Culture, remember, thrives on controlling us through guilt and fear. By stigmatizing our choices, culture engenders so much terror in us that we end up not taking action in the ways we intuitively know to take.

Because we live in a patriarchy, women's choices to fight against stigma are more constrained. The way we dress is stigmatized, as is how we behave, our tone of voice, our choice of words, our sexuality, and the fact that we have a career. If we like sex or don't, want to have children or not, work a lot or not enough, we face judgment along the way. It's easy to see how abuse and divorce are seen by many as taboo.

The stigma of divorce signifies a failure and keeps many women in unhappy and, often, abusive relationships. There is a strong stigma around the label "abused," almost as much as there is around the label "divorcee." It's sad to note that often the ones we feel most judged by are other women. We fear being labeled stupid, incompetent, and immature. This is often why we are reluctant to tell our sisters or mothers about what's happening.

Culture has made us so ashamed of enduring any sort of dysfunction within a marriage that we stay silent. The way we gaslight ourselves is by pretending that bad things are not happening. Instead of holding others responsible, we stay passive in an endless cycle of self-blame. Blaming ourselves is a desperate attempt to gain control of our increasingly uncontrollable outer reality. Instead of creating bolder action-oriented choices, such as honoring our boundaries or exiting the relationship if we are not respected, we stay stuck in a passive attempt to gain control. We imagine all sorts of ways we could be different, believing versions of, "If I hadn't raised my voice, maybe he or she wouldn't act this way toward me."

Calling dysfunction, toxicity, or abuse by their names is the only way to change our reality, whether we are married or not. By calling maltreatment what it is, we empower ourselves to say no and start creating a path to victory. Naming our dysfunction doesn't make us weak. On the contrary, by calling our abusive reality what it is, we diffuse the power it has over us and begin to transcend its limitations.

If you are reading this and are realizing that you have been living a life where you aren't honored, it's time to pick up the phone and call someone, either a friend or a professional. It's time to share your experiences for what they are, without embellishment or self-blame. When you do, you begin to take the reins into your own hands.

The awakened woman understands that her sons, brothers, and male partners face stigma, too, especially when they are abused and may need to leave a marriage, which happens to more males than people realize. When an awakened woman raises her sons, she remembers to counteract the harsh messages they might receive from the patriarchy, reminding them to stay in their heart and to honor their authentic self.

A Transformed Paradigm of Marriage

When marital vows are conducted under the auspices of conscious awareness—where two people love each other in a transcendent way, fully aware of the present-moment quality of their partnership—they have a different quality and energy to them. Rather than binding them to the other forever, each can declare themselves bound to authenticity, growth, and truth. Rather than making promises about the future, they make promises for the present moment. Rather than declaring how they will show up for each other in the future, they commit to first showing up for themselves and honoring themselves in the here and now.

Vows spoken out of inner wholeness celebrate a couple's freedom to choose to stay in love or leave in love. The vows we make are to keep one's own authenticity alive above all else. Here, each understands that as long as growth and honesty are the foundation, all else will fall into place. They realize that the marriage first and foremost reflects their deepest truth, purpose, and authentic selves. Both parties commit to supporting the other on their path of ascendancy, promising not to stand in the other's way and celebrating the other's direction even if it takes them on a different course.

Divorce under this revolutionary new paradigm is a game changer. It looks nothing like the old way, where there was a separation of heart and spirit. On the contrary, it's seen as nothing more than a transformation. Divorce is not a separation from the other person or the family but a movement away from what no longer serves the emerging self. Duality and separation are replaced by interdependence and a unification in which both are free to be true to themselves. There is no winner or loser here. The only outcome is the greater good of everyone. Each person's win is every person's win.

In this model, there is no question of who will "get" the children or where the children will live. Neither is there a dispute over how much money each deserves. Such questions fall by the wayside. The stability of the unit supersedes the stability of any one person. There is no such thing as my lawyer or your lawyer, or my property or yours. The consciousness with which we enter our marriage heavily predicates how we exit the marriage. When we marry with an expanded and transformed consciousness, divorce is conducted under a new consciousness. Everything is shared and held as communal property, only loaned or borrowed for a period of time by one or the other.

An expanded consciousness around marriage understands that it is a life partnership based on respect and the sovereignty of each person in the relationship. By life partnership, I mean it honors and respects the life of each person rather than meaning it lasts for life. It is understood that the legalities are not binding or restrictive. A conscious divorce then requires meditation more than mediation. It is a coming together of two individuals rather than a coming apart. Only this time, they will walk in different directions rather than toward the same horizon.

When we see divorce through these lenses, everything changes. Ego dissolves and spirit rises. The new paradigm of divorce is a release, a surrender, and a return to grace. It constitutes a renewal and a regeneration, not the end. It is not a death but an emergence. It is the dawn of a new era.

15

The Lies About Our Sexuality

Sex is dirty, unchaste, slutty, and shameful
Only to be done with rules and regulations
Anything out of the lines is lewd and obscene
Cloistered and closeted, we inhibit and prohibit
And take what could be divine into the realm of the guttural.

Please don't talk about sex," Tania begged me before I got on stage. I was about to speak to an audience that she claimed was highly religious and therefore potentially prudish.

"You know that I may not be able to avoid these topics given that I am talking on parenting," I warned her.

Not one to give up, she almost threatened me by saying, "Well, if you do, then beware their wrath. This is an uptight audience."

Unafraid of breaking taboos, I went on stage and, within a few minutes, I told the audience what Tania had said about them—without mentioning her name, of course. I immediately felt them tighten up. A few laughed nervously. You would think I was talking to a group of nuns or, worse still, a group of middle schoolers. Perhaps even middle schoolers would be better able to handle these topics than this audience filled with scores of thirty- to seventy-year-olds.

Poor Tania! Little did she realize that her forewarning would lead me to an actual direct confrontation with the one thing she was trying to avoid. We spent the rest of the workshop deconstructing why exactly the audience was so petrified of sex. And do you know what happened? People opened up about their repressive backgrounds, their strict Catholic upbringing, and their shame around their bodies. Many of them said they were talking about sex in the open for the first time in their lives.

The ambience began to lighten up. People became comfortable and everyone's body language became more relaxed. Stories were exchanged, tears were shed, and a new narrative around sex emerged. Unbeknownst to Tania, she was responsible for spearheading a mini-revolution that night, one that every single person in the audience would carry in their hearts forever.

This audience was not the first I had addressed who were uncomfortable around the topic of sex. It's a universal phenomenon. I am no longer surprised at the discomfort adult men and women face when I bring up the topic of sexuality, let alone talk about vaginas, penises, and orgasms. I can see faces grimace, skin flush, and hands flit nervously. Even though I am addressing adults, many act like children, unable to tolerate any talk around these topics. I have sympathy for them, not judgment. I get it. I know how oppressive our conditioning around sex is. It's just a tragedy that we can't talk about the most basic of intimate acts in a transparent way.

It's through sex that each one of us came into the world. Sex is probably one of the most primal and basic instincts we have. An unstoppable force between all animals, it's what makes the world go 'round. Even though sex is natural, normal, and healthy, culture has taken our most organic and authentic expression of self and managed to pervert it into something we need to feel ashamed of. Culture has psychologically manipulated us into believing that loving our bodies and each other's bodies is a bad thing.

We have serious hang-ups around the penis and the vagina, even though they are organic to our bodies—no different than our nose or our fingers. It's laughable. We have even more hang-ups about whose penis enters which vagina. Not only this, we also have heavily crafted stories around masturbation and self-pleasure. How can touching ourselves in the privacy of our own space be something to frown on? When we step back and neutrally dissect each protest at its core, we can surely see how ridiculous it is. We are human and sexual, so what's the hang-up really about?

The sexual act, when conducted in a mutually respectful relationship, has the potential to be full of energy, vitality, power, and passion. It's the most natural, unconditioned energy we possess. Yet the taboos around it make one think it's the most unnatural part of us. To regulate sexuality and inhibit this vital channel of human connection and pleasure is to cut off the life source from life itself.

Do you think that it may be time to ask, What's the big deal about sex?

Let's Talk About Sex, Baby!

Sex is the proverbial elephant in the room—the bedroom, in this case. When we pretend it isn't powerful and yet are ruled by its forceful tide, we create an inner schism. It's akin to losing a loved one to death and acting like we have no grief. Where do these powerful feelings go? What are the repercussions of such constant suppression?

A culture that censures the most vital parts of our essence will pay a heavy price. When things are suppressed without conscious awareness and are shoved into the underworld of our psyche, they don't disappear. They spring from hiding when we least expect them and, like a wildfire, burn everything in their path.

The repercussions of our sexual suppression are profound. If we cannot even talk about sex and body parts, we cannot share. If we cannot share, we cannot learn. If we cannot learn, we cannot grow. If we cannot grow, we cannot integrate. If we cannot integrate, these areas of our lives remain forever split off.

Sex is not only something we can't talk about—it's not even allowed to exist as part of our consciousness. Let's pause for a moment to metabolize just how much inauthenticity this must breed in us. We talk about teaching our children how to deal with feelings as an attempt to raise them with a high social-emotional quotient, but here we are as adults, cut off from an essential conversation about one of the most basic primal forces in our life. It's no wonder most of us are walking around heavily medicated and anxious.

It isn't just women who suffer from this suppression—our children do too. The Catholic church is an example of how acute suppression leads to acute perversion against the weak and vulnerable. Everyone suffers when we deny ourselves authentic sexual expression. I am not condoning the violent and perverse acts that are done in the name of sexuality, but I am certainly asking why these things happen. Why do so many men, and to some degree women, engage in these acts of sexual aggression? I am interested in understanding why so many participate. What led them to this place? What are we doing as a collective that allows sexual aggression to occur?

I was raised in a rigid, primitive, and stringent cultural indoctrination around female sexuality. In my culture, to desire sex—let alone ask for sex or invite it—is considered wanton. It's simply not done. I played out this suppression in my relationships, leading to many arguments and standoffs. As every woman knows, if the emotional environment is not conducive, her sexuality will not reach its peak. When a woman reveres herself and engages in relationships of mutual reverence, her sexuality has no choice but to blossom. We are sexual beings who are repressed due to cultural tyranny. Once that lid is blown off, everything else flows.

Honoring the Animal in Us

Humans are animals. Not *part* of the animal kingdom but animals, period. How is this admission related to our sexuality? By denying we *are* animals, we place ourselves in a superior position to them. We see them and the things they typically engage in, such as primal sexual instincts, as inferior. This is why many of us often refer to our male partners as being "animals" when they are sexually lustful, as if this was a bad thing. The truth is that they are being animals *not* because this is a bad thing but because humans *are* animals. When we enter this awareness, there is no shaming of our primal instincts but, instead, an expanded consciousness around them.

The idea that we are better than animals has its roots in the Bible. Some may be offended by what I write, but if they allow for some open-mindedness, they might see a valid point. The creation story perpetuated by the book of Genesis is that God created this entire universe in seven days. Further, by creating man on the sixth day—the last day, after creating the other "lower" creatures—it suggests that man was God's crowning jewel, created to rule over the rest of the species. Then, to top off the entire saga, it states that God created the woman out of the rib of man.

This story is a blatant denial of the role of evolution. When we tell our children a story that takes us out of the natural order of the universe, we are doing more than entertaining them. We are actually embedding a worldview in their minds, one that strips them of understanding their interconnectedness and oneness with all living beings. Is it any wonder, then, that we now face an unprecedented climate crisis? The reason we can plunder the earth and destroy its diverse creatures is because we truly don't see ourselves as part of its ecosystem. We believe we are better. This attitude of superiority is fully supported in Genesis.

By not understanding just how animal we are, we have moved far away from our authentic truth into a terrain of psychological, cultural, and spiritual degeneration. In order to fully realize our human potential, we need to snap out of our denial that we are not animals. We are human animals, animals in human form. There is great beauty in thinking of ourselves as part of the natural kingdom.

I repeat, we didn't just come *from* animals—we *are* animals. This sub-tle shift of emphasis has a huge psychological impact on us sexually.

Wanting to have sex is not just for "the animals." It is a vital part and parcel of who we are. We are not subhuman for being who we can't help being. Many wisdom gurus talk about transcending our sexuality through abstinence as if transcendence equals austerity and abnegation. The more "spiritual" you are, the less need for sex you are supposed to have. They, too, perpetuate a misguided ap-proach to sex, which only serves to further suppress it.

In my personal experience, this couldn't be further from the truth. I have found that the more "spiritually awakened" I be-come, the more sexually awakened I become. The more my wis-dom blossoms, the more my sexuality does too. As I enter into a more integrated emotional synchrony with myself, this directly leads to a sexual synchrony. Sex is no longer something I do or perform but is an outpouring of who I intrinsically am. The more I feel one with myself and the universe, the more I feel one with my sexuality.

The conscious approach to our sexuality fully integrates it into our daily awareness and conversations. It sees sexuality as natural and organic. It removes the dogma, judgment, and shame around it. By infusing our primal desires with a present-moment con-sciousness, it actually injects the wild with the wise. By allowing our sexuality to be part of our conscious awareness, rather than hidden and suppressed in the shadowy dungeons of our uncon-sciousness, we bring it into higher consciousness. At that point, we can talk about our desires freely and learn how to manage them with discernment, sharing strategies and tools with one another. Bringing sexuality out of the closet is a huge step toward a trans-formed relationship with our primal desires.

Culture has taught us to own others in relationships, particularly their sexual fidelity. Once someone is in a relationship with us, we presume sexual ownership over them. We not only want to possess their hearts but also their sexual organs. Where these organs go is very much our business. You may fear that such a transparent and honest approach toward sex may result in indiscriminate and wild orgies where disease spreads like wildfire. We justify this manic possessiveness by talking about disease control. But we know deep down that it's not about safety as much as "this belongs to me and is off-limits to anyone else." Ownership, possession, and control are the crux of the matter.

When we open up the topic of sexuality and bring it out into the light of day, the secrecy fades, the lies and duplicity become unnecessary, and the capacity for conscious discernment increases. Talking about sex in an open way takes away its mystique. We treat it as it always should have been treated, with natural joy, delight, and a whole lot of loving pleasure.

Conscious sexuality is not about indiscriminate or impulsive acting out. It is fully aware, highly discerning, and completely present to reality. It acts with compassion and responsibility, taking into account the needs of all involved. Far from being exploitative or self-absorbed, it's highly attuned to the evolution of others, passionately invested in the betterment of all.

Our task is to unleash ourselves from the cultural dogma that has subjugated us for eons. These pages are an ode to our intense and immense capacity for sexual and emotional connection, as well as an invitation to break down our taboos.

Thou Shalt Suffer

Our bodies are ours to know. They constitute a portal to the present moment, a way of transcending thought. Grounding ourselves in our body, including our sexuality, allows us to move away from our mental loops and enter the here and now in an embodied way.

Our primary opportunity as humans is to know ourselves. As in all other aspects of our being, self-knowledge—or in this case, sex-knowledge—is the key to relating consciously to the world beyond ourselves. To not know ourselves at the level of our own body is to never fully know the world outside of us. By hiding our own sexuality from ourselves, we infantilize ourselves. By not knowing our own way around town, we give the map to someone else and complain when they cannot steer us in the right direction and we end up lost.

Sister to sister, if we cannot own that we harbor strong and shameful taboos around sexuality, we will never be able to come out of the closet. Ask yourself, What are my true feelings around my sexuality? How well do I really know the folds and crevices of my vagina? Do I truly find myself sexy? What are my fantasies, especially if there was no price to pay? What parts of my sexuality am I suppressing?

In order for us to evolve and elevate ourselves as a species, we must ask what our true fear of sex is really about. Why are we so afraid of two (or more) people enjoying their bodies and expressing their sexual pleasures? Aren't we most loving and calm during sex? The act itself is just simple, isn't it? So the only thing that appears to be wrong is how we look at it. It's here that we have the power to evolve.

Suffering is a motif that runs through much of religion and is enshrined in much of our cultural lore. We are conditioned to believe that the more we suffer, the more we will live chaste lives that will earn our spot in the afterworld.

Most religions, especially the monotheistic ones, indoctrinate us with the idea that we should be ashamed of self-pleasure. These teachings have a defined and prescriptive psychological impact on young minds. When we are conditioned to think that we are inherently faulty by virtue of being alive, we develop a particular psychology of fear around our authentic power, and a deep shame around our self-perceived unworthiness. We don't feel as if we have a right to pleasure or to even be here on this earth. We are made to dissociate ourselves from a direct access to the universe, the earth, and our body. We live in a strangely disconnected and disengaged way.

When religion staked its claim on marriage, it naturally corralled sex also. When marriage began to be considered holy, so did sex within the marriage, whereas sex outside the marriage became unholy. The message this sent was that sex was so bad, it first had to be sanctified by God. Then alone could it be entered into "purely." Sex no longer was something natural and organic but became part of the story of "good and evil." Whenever we are about to have sexual fun, we imagine a God with a stern look uttering, "Thou shalt not."

Religion and many spiritual teachers have us believing in the power of sexual celibacy. This is a cultural story intended to keep us in a state of infantilism, suppression, and disconnection from the power of our body. By cutting us off from the pleasures of our body, we are kept in a state of childlike suppression. The fact is that if women are not *sex*-actualized, we may never be able to be *self*-actualized.

Sexuality by its nature is antisuffering. It is full of pleasure, a celebration at the highest levels. Do you see how our religious natures and our sexual natures clash? It's little wonder that sex scares us. It demands we abandon suffering and enter into our primal nature. Conditioned to believe that suffering is noble, it's little wonder that sex tends to have so much guilt attached to it.

The reason we feel ashamed of sex is because it is the most dramatic example of the universal life force being used for our personal pleasure. Whether pleasuring ourselves through masturbation or sex with another, we declare that we are worthy of joy. We have been taught that this is self-absorbed and selfish, something to feel guilty about. Using the universal life force in a manner that is so highly personal and pleasurable makes us extremely self-conscious. It triggers all kinds of guilt. Are we really supposed to enjoy ourselves this much?

It's no wonder that a great deal of sex is disconnected, robotic, and passionless. We don't know what it means to be integrated in our body and use it for pleasure. On the one hand, much of sex is timid, half-hearted, and seriously lacking in passion while, on the other, it's abusive to the nth degree. Bodies may be entwining, but the heart isn't in it. We don't know how to love with our whole being freely, openly, and, most of all, consciously.

Sex is regulated, not due to disease or pregnancy prevention but due to freedom prevention. Frowning on sex is a way to control people from enacting their intrinsic right to autonomy, joy, privacy, and freedom. By creating legal limits and moral restrictions, culture interferes in the lives of consenting adults and controls them. Through shame, mostly, millions of adults suppress their sexual energy for the sake of fitting in and belonging. If sex weren't regulated and restricted, we would see our authentic nature at play.

Would most couples stay together if both had the choice to choose other sexual partners? Should couples stay together simply because it's a legal requirement to do so? Are there other ways to keep the relationship intact even if the sexual relationship flounders? Should marriage preclude sex with other partners? These are vital questions that need to be examined in order to reach a new understanding of intimacy and sexuality.

So how does sexual emancipation fit into this? Well, any kind of emancipation is a threat to the religious order. And carnal emancipation? The greatest threat of all. Because of its potential to be rhapsodic and delightful, it's seen as too beguiling and intoxicating. The drugged effect of religious indoctrination faces the threat of being replaced by a far more potent drug. Therefore, the institution has ensured that it conditions us from a young age to disconnect from our sexuality.

Sexual autonomy and freedom go against the ideal that religion has drilled into us—that we are to live in submission, subservience, sacrifice, and shame. To live in unabashed pleasure, Dionysian in our claim to ecstasy, flies directly in the face of the religious ideal of deference to an external force outside ourselves.

Dismantling Monogamy

Andrea, one of my clients, burst into tears in the middle of the session. She sobbed so hard I thought she was going to choke. I knew something was drastically wrong. This was a woman who rarely showed any emotion. "I think George is having an affair. I saw some texts on his phone. What am I going to do?" She had been married for fifteen years. Her kids were twelve and seven. What was she going to do indeed?

As we kept talking, her tears gave way to anger. "I am furious with him. Here I am, slogging away at home, taking care of the kids, the cooking, and the laundry. And this is how he repays me? By sleeping with some secretary at his office? What am I, chopped liver?" Andrea was hurt and felt rejected. This is normal. After all, she was scared. Like many women do, she had given up her full-time job when she gave birth and was now dependent on her husband for money.

Andrea and I worked for an entire year on her ideas around monogamy and infidelity. She and her husband entered couples therapy with another therapist and are still working out their issues. The reason I brought up her story in this introduction is to highlight one of the most common problems faced by couples: infidelity.

Infidelity is one of the leading causes of marital disruption and divorce. Because the idea of "sacred marriage" comes with monogamy, having sex with anyone outside marriage is considered downright sacrilegious and illegal, sometimes even punishable by death.

Monogamy implies that our sexual desire must be confined to just one body for the rest of our lives. If one strays, it is considered the darkest type of betrayal against a partner and grounds for divorce. I couldn't even begin to count the number of marriages that have broken up due to infidelity, mostly on the part of the man. Women have been fully conditioned to believe that monogamy is the only way to love and be loved. Men want to believe this story, too, but their libidinal needs often cause them to act the opposite. Like in Andrea's case, the woman in such instances endures unmitigated strife and suffering.

The onus is on women because, more than men, we have fully bought into the story around monogamy and suffer the most as a result. While many women cheat, it is clear from the data that more men cheat than women when dating and within marriage. Whether at the level of fantasy, porn, or actual physical inter-course, most men have expressed or acted on their sexual desires outside their primary relationship. This fact has led many a woman to feel betrayed, confused, and hurt. While I am not advocating that a man lie or "cheat," men are biologically wired for variety. By being imbued with the ambition to spread their seed, most male animals are wired for promiscuity. Why do you think some men want their women to dress in lingerie or watch porn during sex? It's because seeking variety is part of their nature. While this behavior could be objectifying in some cases, in other cases it could just be a man's safer way of fulfilling his desire for variety and novelty. How do we women typically respond to such demands? We are often outraged, indignant, righteous. We may immediately take things personally and feel betrayed. We are inclined to degrade the man and his love as lesser-than and want to leave the relationship.

As for the men? They are often befuddled by our intense re-action. For them, sex is often "just" sex and biological relief. For women, it's more about love, loyalty, and ethics. It's here that men and women differ the most, fight the most, and lose the most.

Men's sexuality is intricately related to their biology. Women's is more related to their psychology. This means women have bought into culture's stories around sex way more than men have. If we are not willing to own our judgment and emotion around sex, we won't be able to meet men where they are and, in this regard, will forever be hurt for no good reason. If we learned how to be open about sex and understood a man's libidinal nature, we would separate sexual relief from love, and change our narrative around monogamy.

When we are more aware of the inherent sexual differences be-tween males and females, we open ourselves up to new realities. Were our partners to then want to watch pornography or introduce another person into the sexual dyad, we wouldn't throw ourselves into a tizzy. Our men would feel safe to talk to us about their in-nermost desires and needs, in this way ending the need to lie and cheat behind our backs. We would stop playing mommy to them or to their conscience and instead enter a true adult-to-adult partnership with them.

I must clarify again, I am not for pornography or nonmonogamy per se. Neither am I against them. I am simply making a case about our lack of choice around them, and our judgment and fear of them. Sure, the porn industry has major flaws, such as exploitation and degradation of women, that need to be severely reconstructed and I am fully against women being objectified and treated as sex slaves. Yet many men are drawn to porn sites only for viewing and masturbatory pleasure. Instead of denigrating these men for these compulsions, we need to understand them. Failing to create a bridge toward them, we will engender an even greater abyss between the sexes.

Countless women have come to me in sessions complaining about their partners needing to watch pornography during sex, making the women feel insecure and lesser-than. When I explain to these women that they have been indoctrinated to feel this way, they often breathe a sigh of relief. When I explain to them how their male partners are wired for this kind of extra stimulation and that it is not personal against them, they relax. By opening our minds to this hot topic without the heat of judgment and emotion, we go a long way in bringing ourselves closer to our male counterparts.

In any group of men and women, it's the men who are far more able to be honest and open about their sexuality. Most women cannot even articulate what their sexual needs are, let alone ways they could get them met. Unless this mental barrier around sexuality changes, our men will not be able to speak candidly about their sexuality, and we will lose the deep connection we could otherwise have. If someone chooses to be more sexually active, creative, or polygynous, stepping beyond their primary relationship for sexual gratification, does this mean they are automatically bad?

Before Western imperialism, 83 percent of indigenous societies were polygynous, with 16 percent monogamous, and 1 percent polyandrous (where a woman has more than one husband). Nature built us for connection and sexuality without the dogma and prescriptions found in religion. It gave us the tools for sexual intimacy and pleasure without rules and convention, ritual, or ceremony. Like all the other animals who are more in tune with their nature, connection and sexual relationships were sorted under the auspices of the collective tribe, who somehow found an equilibrium through polygyny.

My challenge isn't that we should abandon monogamy but that we understand that it, like most institutions, is constructed by culture. It is not our natural way. And because of this, it should be a choice.

We must disrupt the implicit marriage between morality and monogamy if we are to have honest conversations around sexuality. Religions propagate the idea that monogamy is the only "pure" way. As such, we associate it with "goodness." When someone then strays, we consider them "bad." Actually, scratch that. We associate them with the devil himself. And it is here, in this marriage between religion, morality, and monogamy that we have inculcated archaic views around our sexuality, which then cause immeasurable and unnecessary suffering. Our sexuality is an expression of the wildest and most untamed part of our essence. To steal that part of us and condition it with heavy-duty fear and shame is a tragedy. It's as if our power has been castrated, denying us access to joy and bliss—mass control at its finest.

Nature gave women the capacity to nurture their young and partake in relationships, but it didn't ask us to be the be-all and end-all for just one man, nor one man to be all things for one woman. Nature didn't speak in terms of twin souls and soulmates. Nature is not ethereal or romantic but is, instead, practical. It lives in the actual experience and practice of life, not in the hypothetical. Ask men and women in a monogamous dyad about their sexual compatibility and I guarantee that their answers will resound with complaints. In my past relationships, we constantly argued about our differing sexual needs. While my male partner, whoever it was at the time, could have sex once or more every twenty-four hours, I was happy with once a week. As a result, either he or I compromised in some way. Nature knows that because males across species generally want more sex than females, polygyny and nonmonogamy are options. If we don't allow this and instead force the male to stay with one woman for his primary sexual gratification in perpetuity, there will likely be a high degree of sexual frustration. This dissonance is not just due to imbalances in libido but also due to the long periods of reduced female sexual availability—i.e., menses, last trimester of pregnancy, postpartum periods, and postmenopause.

Instead of understanding that the rules of monogamy are themselves false, we beat ourselves to a pulp and believe ourselves unworthy and defective for having any desire for sexual exploration outside our primary partnership. We believe there is something wrong with us or our partner and either discard the intimate relationship altogether by vilifying the other, or we contort ourselves to look more desirable, believing this will keep the other from straying.

On the man's side, he is often castigated and denigrated in public for following his libidinal needs. The onslaught of shame and blame we inflict on each other over infidelity has subverted our understanding of his biological underpinnings. The person is excoriated for his actions, as well as for lying, then sent to the guillotine without ever having the chance to educate, or be educated, about why they acted in these ways and what they can do to harness their sexual energy. Of course, this can be true for women as well, but I focus on men here because the preponderance of cases of infidelity are often instigated by them.

The actual crux of the matter isn't who is the initiator of infidelity but instead something far more basic: how can we be honest about our sexual desires and preferences within and outside of the marriage? One can barely even explore these topics hypothetically. Sometimes a partner is just trying to "check things out," so that they can clear their own confusions. Even this act is considered bad. Of course, the ideal is that one doesn't have any desires outside of the dyad. But is this realistic? Can we expect every dyad to be perfectly aligned? What if one in the couple needs space to explore their sexuality in a different way? Unless this space is consciously created, trust is eroded and lovers end up as enemies.

We are so indoctrinated into monogamy that it is hard to believe we can exist without it. The idea that we should be pair-bonded with the opposite sex in an exclusive relationship for the rest of our lives is embedded in our psyche. Yet when we allow ourselves to step back for a moment and understand that monogamy is a recent cultural invention that goes against our innate biological nature, we can revisit our ideas around it and allow for an expanded consciousness.

I know this is hard for women to hear. Before my own spiritual renaissance, it would have been hard for me to hear too. I would have scoffed and scornfully thought, "This is total nonsense. Men need to grow up and stop acting like horny teenagers!" We see their lust as immature and infantile. And while we could be right in that many men exhibit their sexuality in impulsive ways, we need to understand how culture, and women as part of this culture, have helped cocreate this unconscious acting out on their part.

Most men do not know how to handle their sexual wiring. It's a significant issue for most of them. Their minds become cloudy and their focus gets lost. Their sexuality impedes clear discernment. You may think I am making excuses for them. Far from it—I am trying to understand them.

Once again, I am not speaking about sexual violence or toxic sexopathy. I am talking about a consciously awakened sexuality—one that allows for honesty. Just as we crave understanding for our emotional needs, men crave understanding for their sexual needs. We women first need to feel connected before we have sex, whereas they need have sex to feel connected. For us, connection is the pathway to sex and for them it is the opposite. It is just the way each is wired. When both in the couple awaken to what matters to them and are able to communicate this in an honest way, they bridge their differences rather than create more distance.

Don't get me wrong. Women also have the capacity to be nonmonogamous and should feel absolutely free and safe to explore this in their own right. What if a woman is attracted to another male outside her marriage or is discontented with her husband's libido or sexual prowess? Should she be made to feel slutty and like a whore if she wishes to fulfill herself with another human, male or female? Women need to feel empowered to speak of their sexual desires and fantasies. No woman should feel sexually caged just because she is married. Sadly for us, the current sexual standards keep both of us feeling ashamed for wanting to seek sexual pleasure outside our relationship. This needs to change. It all begins with our own awakening. The more each of us awakens from within, the more we will hold space for enlightened sexual exchanges on the outside. The more liberated we are in our views, freeing ourselves from religion's puritanical hold on us, the more men and women can feel guilt free and shame free to explore their sexuality.

Redefining the "Cheater"

When we use the label "cheater," we are typically referring to a man. The reason for this is that men are more likely than women to cheat.

I want us to go beyond blame and shame to seek what lies beneath this near-universal phenomenon. In order to understand a man, we need to begin our quest by asking the right question: Why has culture put men in a box when nature set them up wanting to break out of it? The box is the cage of monogamy. If nature made its males inherently polygynous, culture's imposition of monogamy goes directly against her directive.

I know this may bring up severe reactions for many women who have been cheated on. I invite you to pause and know that I am not diminishing your pain. What I am trying to show you is that the reason this pain exists is because we have been set up to feel it.

We aren't the only ones who feel this pain. Men who wish to act on their sexual desires outside their primary relationship know they cannot do so because of the way society frowns on it. They know that they only have two choices—to suppress their needs or engage in duplicitous behavior and suffer the shame of having done so. Whenever I ask men who have engaged in "cheating" if it was their conscious will, each of them said it wasn't. A common complaint was that they felt they couldn't confide in their partners about their desires and needs and that they wished they could. They each admitted that had they been able to share their feelings with their partners authentically, they might not have felt the need to veer off on their own.

Instead of vilifying men, we can bring ourselves into a conscious awareness of how their biology affects them. By allowing an open dialogue around sexuality, we no longer allow perversions to grow in dark closets. If boys were taught at a young age to treat their sexuality with a conscious awareness and weren't shamed, they wouldn't later feel the need to prey upon young bodies or vulnerable females. They would be able to speak of their inner longings and conflicts openly and seek the help they need to integrate their experiences into their emotional repertoire.

By talking about the effects of monogamy on men's psyches and, more importantly, how they deal with an individual female's sex drive—which is often considerably lower than theirs—we help men get a handle on their sexual fantasies and how this plays into their day-to-day lives with a monogamous partner.

If we judge our men constantly, how can we show them that we care about them as much as we want them to care about us? Once we open the door for men to share their sexual needs, interests, curiosities, and desires in an open and honest way, we can embrace unions that go beyond transactions, ownership, possession, and control.

The channel for an enlightened and open dialogue around male sexuality (and female sexuality) is sorely missing. When we give it space to exist, we allow men's sexual demons to exit the closet. By harnessing their libidinal energy more consciously, they move away from their customary role of aggressive sexual predators to compassionate lovers of women—ones who respect and honor women's boundaries as much as they sexually desire such women.

When was the last time you heard a man tell his wife, "I would like to have sex with your friend" or "I have a sexual fantasy about a woman at work that I need to work through with you"? Probably never. There would be harsh repercussions for such talk. We don't need to be taught to stay away from such topics. We intuitively know that these are not for the realm of everyday dinner conversations.

"But he took a vow and is a liar!" many women bemoan. Religion has us taking vows of eternal fidelity at the time of marriage. When we break these vows, we feel terrible guilt. We are blamed for being sinners and liars. The truth is that the whole concept of "taking a vow" is faulty in the first place. As discussed earlier, how can a young person, still largely unconscious, be held accountable to a promise for the rest of their lives?

I cannot tell you how many people I have met who feel sexual energy toward others outside their primary relationship and have no way to process their feelings. The cost of telling the truth is too high. The person meting out the cost is part of this dynamic. Safety in a relationship is created by both parties and is never a one-sided job. When we create the atmosphere for transparent authenticity, we actually become more intimate than we ever thought possible. In fact, the greatest intimacy and connection emerges when we are honest—first with ourselves, then with each other.

Onto a New Sexual Terrain

We don't realize how our culture's set ways stifle our authentic voice. When we understand how nature intended us to be versus how our culture conditioned us to be, we set ourselves free. Until then we will be bound by invisible chains.

The truth is that conscious relationships can exist in all sorts of configurations. It is up to us to decide what formation works best for our emotional and sexual needs. Culture, via religion, created one supposedly "right" way so that it could control our freedom to choose what best suits us. By industrializing our sexuality, it put us in a factory line and organized us in robotic patterns. This way, we couldn't create our own way of life. By regimenting our sexuality through fear and control, culture tamed our wild sexuality and slowly annihilated it into an insipid version of its original form.

Consciousness and awakened intimacy involve moving beyond the paradigm of fear and separation into a new dimension of transparency and cooperation. We don't own anyone and no one owns us. Consciousness demands that we engage in tough but crucial conversations that allow each in the relationship to be introspective and transparent about their needs and desires. Only through this kind of open sharing can partners reach their highest potential. For this to happen, we need to create the space to ask the questions most couples avoid:

> Are we sexually and emotionally compatible?
> What are our sexual fantasies and desires?
> How can we sexually improve to meet each other's needs?
> Are we both bringing our truest selves to the fore, or are we hiding parts of ourselves from each other?
> Are we creating an atmosphere of safety such that transparency, diversity, and truth can be shared without judgment or shame?

When we create the space for honest inquiry, we signal to the other person that we are invested in their inner exploration. We allow for transparency to exist that otherwise would not. Let's take a stereotypical scenario. A man in a relationship begins to feel sexually dissatisfied. While his wife is at work, he begins to look at porn to satisfy his urges. Soon he begins to visit strip clubs with his male friends. One day, he meets another woman and engages in sex. Do you know what kind of hell is going to break loose in his home? The wife will never understand her husband's sexual nature. She will feel destroyed and will possibly end their relationship. Of course, women are not exempt from this kind of pattern either. This kind of behavior abounds in both sexes and in all kinds of relationships.

The conscious way asks, What need is this person trying to meet? If I cannot meet this need, how can we arrange for it to be met through other means? How am I not showing up for this person in a manner that allows them to thrive? Do I care enough to change the dynamic so I can meet this person's needs?

Do you see how different the conscious and awakened approach is to the traditional approach? If the couple decides that the future is unsustainable, they can agree to part. When things are seen through the vantage of cocreation, no one feels like the bad guy, and certainly no one is treated like a pariah.

To illustrate how this works in everyday life, Carolina, one of my clients, came to me after her six-month-long affair had been discovered by her husband, Derek. Their twenty-four-year marriage was being threatened by this infidelity. More than Derek, though, it was Carolina who was most wound up and traumatized by her sexual dalliance.

Carolina came to me to fix herself, as she put it. Distraught and unhinged, Carolina was guilt-ridden and self-shaming. "I never thought I would be the one who would be so bad. I never thought I could stoop so low. I am a terrible person!" The only way I could help her get over her infidelity—and it took a long time—was to help her realize that it wasn't connected to her morality. I slowly led her to see that she had not cheated on anyone and, if anything, had been cheating herself out of her own fulfillment in the marriage.

Carolina and Derek decided to build on their marriage. They began to see that each had different sexual and emotional needs from the other and an affair was not necessarily the end of the relationship, but a pointer that something needed healing. Carolina began to express herself more authentically and allowed Derek to do the same. They both began the painstaking work of sharing their feelings in a way they had never done before. In this way, their true union finally began.

What would have happened if both had allowed culture's conventions to lead the way? They wouldn't have given each other a chance to discover something deeper and more profound. Theirs is a clear example of how our ideas around cheating can stand in the way of a deeper connection.

So many of us are cheating on ourselves, aren't we? We are living in constant inauthenticity, faking a persona for the world around us. When we don't show up for ourselves or the other in truth, we are, in essence, cheating. This isn't a lesser evil than sexual cheating. It should hold equal weight, if not more. Once we realize we haven't shown up in the relationship as our true self, we might be willing to concede that the other's behavior is not too far off from our own. This enables us to shift to a new way of relating to ourselves and each other. Instead of being destroyed by such behavior, we can grow and evolve through it.

It's time to move away from our conventional understanding of relationships toward a more liberated one, where we release each other from impossible codes of conduct. As we do so, we find out who we are without the fear of being shamed by or abandoned by the other.

Toward a Transcendent Intimacy

Truth be told, *intimacy* is generally a euphemism for *sex*. We are so embarrassed to discuss sex, we colloquially refer to it as intimacy. In reality, much of the sex we have is just copulation. It's hardly intimate, which is precisely why so many wives especially complain about the fact they have to have sex with their husbands. They see it as a chore because, in many ways, it is.

While sex focuses on the form of our bodies in copulatory action, intimacy infuses the sexual experience with the qualities of the transcendent—formless connection and emotional union. Many couples think they are intimate when, in fact, they are just engaging in the act of copulation. Big difference.

Conscious sexuality doesn't begin in our loins. It begins in our minds and hearts, which is where the greatest sex is birthed. When two people are physically attracted to each other, there is a fiery energy that is quite seductive. However, this rarely lasts past the "honeymoon phase" of the relationship. What lasts is the couple's mental and emotional connection. If this isn't strong, then no matter how great the sex is, the intimacy will fade.

The best sex has little to do with what happens between the bedsheets and all to do with what happens when we are out of the bedroom. Lasting sexual connection and rhapsody emerge from a deep emotional and spiritual bond. Sexual chemistry is just one facet of the deeper intimacy couples share. It doesn't imply sensuality and connection at all. To be sensual and connected means to see the other as a mirror, an echo of the best version of the self, where the parts of one are found in the other. The resonance between the two is so profound that the separation that exists between their forms dissolves. Everything they do is sensual because it is deeply connected.

As such, true intimacy goes way beyond sex. Lovemaking happens in unexpected ways and places—in the way two people have dinner together, grocery shop, hold hands on a hike, or tend to their children. Intimacy penetrates every aspect of our lives. It's a reflection of who we are in our most mundane of moments. The more connected we are to our partners during our ordinary life, the more sexual we are in the bedroom. It all begins with how we partner with each other during the day.

True sexual chemistry has nothing to do with how the person looks or how much money they have. Neither is it something we can create only by imbibing chemicals. The real chemistry occurs within us. When we feel connected to the other in a truly intimate way, our body creates its own internal stimulants and psychedelics. When we experience this, we touch upon our innate potential to be sexually transcendent. Deep emotional and spiritual connection is the real aphrodisiac.

In an awakened state, to be intimate means to be *in*-time and *into*-mate. It reflects a deep, ongoing connection with the other in the present moment and in the union with the other. The very word can be broken into *"into-me-see,"* where the "me" is the part of ourselves we see reflected through the mirror of the relationship. Intimacy is about how we integrate and depend on each other, honoring one who honors us and seeing the other within ourselves. Real intimacy forges a bond of oneness and dissolves boundaries of separation. It collectively aggregates all the integral pieces of each partner and merges them into a conscious recognition of the partner as the self.

When we are truly engaging in intimacy, the act of sex is not a verb. It is not an action we take that begins and ends with a goal but is who we intrinsically are. Through our touch during the day, our dialogue, our shared memories, and our spontaneous laughter, it's how we share experiences with each other with abandon and transparency. All these ways translate to how we are in the bedroom.

When a couple moves beyond culture's definitions of sex, they open their relationship up to all sorts of play and spontaneity. They may bring in other partners if they wish, or they may not. The fact is that they have moved beyond the form restrictions of traditional sex and opened themselves up to the emotional connection they feel between themselves and the universe at large. They are no longer confined or constrained. They are a love unit that is love itself, with no separation within themselves or with the universe.

True intimacy between two free and whole adults is borderless, formless, and timeless. It doesn't focus on the form of the human, or the context. It connects to the essence of the other(s) with no judgment, no conditions. When there is real intimacy, we lose ourselves in the awareness that there is no nonintimate time. We are in-time with our mate at all times. Actual clock time then dissolves, and there is no then, only now. The masters of the *Kama Sutra* understood this and some seekers still do. As I have spiritually deepened, I have discovered this elevated intimacy myself, and it has been cathartic and therapeutic for my soul.

No true intimacy with another can occur without intimacy with the self. It's only when we first have a deep inner union that we can foster a union with another. When we can enjoy, accept, and celebrate our own body through masturbatory pleasure, we can begin to unionize with another in a beautiful and loving way. How can we enjoy another's body and consecrate it with presence when we haven't done this for ourselves?

Our sexual energy holds a vitality that is incomparable and indefatigable. When it is uncaged from the boxes and labels of gender, marriage, monogamy, or sexual orientation, it is free—free to *be*.

16

The Lies About Motherhood

Her children are her zenith of achievement
Her medals of glory and pride
Through them she finally feels worthy
Purposeful, zestful, and alive
Without them she feels adrift, empty, and lost.

Do you know of any item on a young woman's bucket list that shows up more consistently than motherhood? Even more than becoming a wife, the desire to be a mother may trump everything else in the life of many women. From the time we play with our little dolls in our make-believe houses, the majority of us dream of having our own children. Becoming a mother feels as second nature to most of us as being female itself. It is a checkbox on many girls' lists, one they believe they "should" check off at all costs. If she chooses not to have children at a later age, she will pay the price of having to explain her motivations ad nauseam to an unforgiving culture.

I still remember when my friend Tricia called me in distress. Her voice was tense and somber. "He doesn't want to have kids!" she said. "How can he not want to be a dad? I thought we were going to start a family." Tricia was thoroughly confused. She had a tinge of judgment in her voice, as if her husband, Stan's, desire not to have kids meant he was selfish. I explained to her that he may not be ready, or that fatherhood wasn't up his alley. Tricia wasn't buying it. Because motherhood to her felt so natural, she just couldn't understand why it wasn't the same for him. She interpreted it as a sign he lacked commitment. No matter how I tried to explain to her that men were wired differently, she was vehement. "This is a game changer, a deal breaker! If he doesn't want to have any kids, I'm out."

For many women like Tricia, motherhood is a game changer and a deal breaker. It is one of their most important goals. It is the dream they have been waiting for, the fantasy they are thirsty to fulfill. Only through the actualization of this goal do many women feel complete.

One of the first cultural lies around motherhood is that it is a "should" and that we are somehow lesser if we choose not to become a mother. While our bodies are wired to conceive and nurture our young, many of us are unable to or decide against it. When this happens, it's imperative for us to realize that culture has created shame around the "nonmother," and it is one of the lies it continues to spread to us.

As I said before, *to mother* doesn't require having a biological child. All women—all humans, actually—have the capacity to embody and enact the mothering function. To believe that the child must come via our own uterus is to endorse a limited view of motherhood. We are all mothers. Once we embrace this reality, we can stand tall in our choices, whether it be to physically birth a child or not.

Should a woman choose to physically birth or adopt a child, she needs to understand that she is about to embark on one of the most profound journeys of her life. There is no more epic a transformation that she is likely to endure than entering motherhood. The psychological transformations a woman goes through on becoming a mother are indeed nothing short of monumental. Ask any mother and she will tell you how gargantuan the shift in consciousness from premotherhood to motherhood was for her. Many women describe this transformation as a death of sorts, where the old parts of her slough off to reveal a brand-new entity within. For many, it's an encounter with parts of themselves they never even knew existed—especially their compassionate, loving, giving, sacrificing, and nurturing parts.

Once a woman becomes a mother, she is irrevocably transformed. Many women have described the feeling of having their heart walk around in the body of their child. A mother often places her children and their well-being before her own. Where before she might have been zealously protective of her space and time, she now knows that neither belong to her in quite the same way. She intuitively understands that she is now a humble but willing vessel her children can drink from, sleep in, and forever know they can come back to. From this moment on, she is no longer a woman in her own right but always and irrevocably someone's mother.

Mirror, Mirror on the Wall

"I knew it was going to be hard, but I didn't realize it would be this hard," Zara sobbed. "I know I am being childish. This is so silly because it's a good thing, but I can't help myself." She had dropped her youngest child, Clint, off for college three weeks ago and was finding the adjustment extremely difficult. "I am so used to being a mother that I just don't know what to do with myself now. He was my baby boy and I know I need to let him be an adult, but I am so scared. To me, he is still a kid."

Zara, like a million moms who experience "empty-nest syndrome," was having an extremely hard time adjusting to her new reality. For the first time, perhaps, she needed to ask herself, "Who am I now?" Throughout all the years we raise our children, we identify as "mother." When that role fades, we are left befuddled about who we are supposed to be.

"Clint has been miserable so far," Zara opined. "He calls me every day and says he wants to come home. I wish he would make new friends and get his life started. I just want him to be happy. If he is happy, I will move on." My task was to help Zara realize that she had placed all sorts of expectations on Clint's adjustment to college and was highly invested in his happiness. Now that he was having a hard time in his early weeks, she was facing a huge inner crisis.

Most mothers will attest that their well-being and sense of worth is inextricably tied to how happy their children are. Motherhood comes with the diagnosis of an extreme and sometimes obsessive codependency. As a line from the movie *Hustlers* states, "Motherhood is a mental illness." This inability to detach is a double-edged sword. On the one hand, attachment comes with the wonderful ability to create lasting and deep bonds. But, on the other hand, if the mother isn't careful, this ability will morph into an unhealthy enmeshment. Many moms give up their careers to raise their kids. This loss of their independent vision for themselves has the potential to create a void within, one they seek to fill through their children.

When a woman identifies with the role of mother and sees it as her next career path, she sees what her children achieve and how they progress as her own "next PhD" or career milestone. The danger of such an enmeshment is that she projects onto her kids many of her own unfulfilled longings, using them to meet her unmet fantasies. Without her conscious awareness, she begins to "create and construct" her children like she would a résumé that reflects her vision for herself more than it does her child's vision.

It's important for women to understand just how powerful our projections are toward our children. This is where my work on conscious parenting comes in. Its main premise is to challenge parents to realize that much of how they act toward their children comes from their own inner longings, desires, and old wounds, and has less to do with their children's actual behavior.

The traditional paradigm of parenting is that parenting is about the child. When the child is the focus, the parent feels free to place all sorts of demands and expectations on them without any awareness of their own agenda or motivation. The conscious parenting paradigm turns this on its head and makes parenting about the parent. The parent is challenged to turn the spotlight on themselves and question how their own childhood and life experiences impact the way they parent.

As we awaken to our inner processes, we begin to see how we use our children to heal and complete parts of ourselves that we left behind in childhood. Only when we are willing to look in the mirror do we see how our relationship with our children reflects back how we need to grow from within. Our motherhood journey now takes an important shift.

Culture has set an archetypal standard for how children "should" be—obedient, compliant, nice, happy, and successful. If they are not, they are not good enough. So whom does this responsibility fall on? The parent—and, in most cases, the mother. If the mother has bought into the cultural script that she was never good enough, then motherhood will trigger this pain repeatedly. The truth is that this standard is not only unattainable, it's false. If we don't awaken to its falsity, we begin to tether our worth to unreachable standards and perpetuate our gnawing and profound sense of unworthiness.

Our children shouldn't have to conform to a standard of excellence based on our ideas. They are born to enact their own destiny according to their unique spirit. Of course, on the way toward this, it's natural to desire that our children should grow up to be kind and civil to others, but how exactly they live their lives is up to them.

As we awaken in our own life and begin to set our authentic selves free, we create the conditions for those with whom we share our lives to do so as well. Where before we might have been unconscious to the ways in which we controlled our children's behavior and moods in order to feel good about ourselves, we are now more conscious of this and try hard to separate our children's path from our own. We begin to go through the process of individuation in our own lives, where we psychologically differentiate between ourselves and our role as mom. We see the two as connected but separate. This is how we eventually come to be with our children as well—connected but separate.

This separation is not a bad thing. Instead, separation is extremely vital for both our own and our children's psychological development. It's the process by which we differentiate between who we are and the roles we play. As we mature in this process, we begin to do what we should have done all along—see our children as deeply interconnected with us but at the same time individuated and differentiated from us. We don't enmesh ourselves with them in the same way. All this occurs only when we stop fusing our essence with the role of mother. As we let go of our investment in the mother role, we enter the deeper aspects of the mothering journey, where we don't mother from our mind with agendas and expectations but, instead, from our heart, where we are deeply invested in one thing only—the authentic unfolding of ourselves and our children.

The Golden Child

If there is one area of our lives where the disease of perfectionism tends to raise its unchecked head, it's in our role as mothers. Motherhood has the potential to take our obsession with goodness to a whole new level. We tend to become perfectionists on steroids. We take our own curse of "the golden woman" and project it onto our innocent children, expecting them to carry our unburned torch to become "the golden child." It's no longer enough that we are beautiful and accomplished—now our children need to be this way too. When they shine, we shine. Do they do well in school? If they don't, this must mean *we* are failures as mothers. Do they love their grandma or their father more than they do us? Well, if they do, this must mean *we* are not very lovable. Do they get depressed or anxious? If so, this must mean *we* are to blame.

Culture has subtly and not so subtly placed inordinate pressures on women to be all-giving mothers. Today's "helicopter mom" got her title because she hovers over the children providing them with all they need, from entertainment to stimulation, education, and, of course, the perfect nutrition. By buying into cultural scripts around perfect motherhood, we allow ourselves to be bullied into endeavoring to be perfect moms. If we fall short, we believe we are "bad" moms and blame ourselves for this shortcoming. Mother-hood then becomes its own tyranny, both for the mother and her kids. We bully ourselves better than culture ever could, and also bully other women into the same shame we feel.

While many mothers opt out of the race to win the Best Mother trophy, there are millions who vie for it, albeit at a subconscious level. We engage in subtle forms of competition against other moms without even necessarily knowing we are doing so. Each time we drop our children off at school dressed to the nines, post pictures of our perfect organic lunchboxes, or talk about our children's stel-lar grades, we engage in a subtle act of bullying. Every time we talk about how we handstitched their Halloween costumes late into the night, or how we threw our kids the most elaborate birthday parties with satin-clad invitations, we engage in comparison and competi-tion. We may be doing so innocently and may not have intention-ally meant anything by sharing these "triumphs," but the fact that we display our accomplishments for strangers begs the question of why. What's the underlying motivation? What's the need?

Why do we post our perfections on social media? Why do we display our children's trophies or their achievements? Sure, we are proud, but the questions still remains, why do we need to display this to others? Is there a part of us that desires to be seen in a certain light? Does it give us a sense of pride to boast about our children, our belongings, or our possessions? As a receiver of these "perfect mommy" posts, I feel a subtle, yet direct, pressure urging me to do better. Instead of banding together as mothers who understand the cultural pressures we face, we pit ourselves against one another. In-stead of posting our follies, foibles, and faux pas, we try to appear perfect. We don't realize how damaging this is not only for others but also for ourselves. We all suffer when we present a false idea of motherhood.

As long as we aspire to provide our children with an A+ life, gleaning our identities from this grade, we will set both ourselves and our kids up for failure. Not only will we constantly compare ourselves to other moms and come up short, we will project this lack onto our children and push them to become the torchbearers of the worth we never felt.

Soon enough, we realize our children are here to manifest their own being and can only be manipulated so much. Before we know it, their budding temperament shows us we have to release control over them. We cannot protect our children from their failures, their breakups, their tragedies, or their rejections. No matter how much we love them or how we raise them, they will face pain—sometimes terrible pain. Once we accept this, we can get back in our own lane and raise our children accepting their clear boundaries and without melding our lane with theirs.

The Holy Grail of Parenthood

"You are only as happy as your least happy child," the saying goes. Most parents quote this to explain their state of malaise and unease around their parenting struggles. After all, if their least happy child is really unhappy, what is a parent to do?

You might be shocked when I say it, but this quote is garbage. It speaks to problematic issues, such as the idea that enmeshment with our children's moods is okay. It also suggests that our happiness can be deeply affected by another's happiness or lack thereof. Society considers it a sign of love and care when we share the same feelings as our children.

Once again, culture has endorsed false ideas that influence us deeply. Only when we begin to deconstruct them do we liberate ourselves and our kids and save ourselves a whole lot of anxiety. Culture has long endorsed two shiny goals for parenthood—our children's happiness and success. Ask any parent what their top two goals are and they will almost unanimously agree, "I want my kid to be happy and successful." Let's deconstruct each of these, beginning with happiness.

Zara, the client of mine who was experiencing empty-nest syndrome, was clear. "Until Clint gets happier, I am going to be miserable. We have always been close. Everything I feel, he feels, and vice versa. Now that he is away, I can't even sleep knowing he's in distress. It's killing me."

Parents actually believe that when we mirror our children's feelings, we are being loving and caring. This couldn't be further from the truth. This is not caring—this is enmeshment. When I explained to Zara that she was in a codependent relationship with her son, she was amazed. Not once had she considered that her bond with him was dysfunctional. As I taught her about codependency and how she had lost her identity in that of her son's, it all began to fall into place. She finally saw how her own inability to handle "big feelings" had stopped him from being able to process his feelings his whole life. She was doing it again with this current transition. Instead of going within and sitting with the emotions this new phase of life was bringing up for her, she was going outward and focusing on Clint's happiness. Instead of allowing him to have his own independent relationship with his transition and giving him the space to process his feelings, she was putting pressure on him to feel happy so that she didn't have to deal with the anxiety of having to confront who she was when she wasn't Mom.

More than this, even, I taught Zara that the goal of having "happy" children is a completely unrealistic, irrational, and ultimately impossible goal. It's actually a setup for the opposite to occur. The more we focus on happiness, the more we will be unhappy. Let me explain.

We have turned happiness into a goal when it's really only an emotion—a fleeting one at that. So attached have we become to the idea of being happy that we foolishly aspire to it to be a standing goal. In this, we subconsciously expect life to keep producing happy states. When life complies, we feel lucky, blessed, and fortunate. When life doesn't follow through, we feel downtrodden and miserable. We blame life when, instead, we should blame our foolish expectations.

Happiness is a transient feeling. It comes and goes, like all feelings. It's not something to be attached to. When we are attached to it, we are eager for our next happy "fix." Subconsciously, we resist and reject those life experiences that cause us any degree of sadness, anger, or pain. Ask yourself, is this a realistic way to live—only wanting a life of rainbows and sprinkles?

The harsh truth of parenthood is that our kids are going to feel pain and there is nothing we can do about it. They are going to struggle, flounder, and fail. They are going to make huge mistakes and enter dysfunctional relationships. They may even harm themselves and their lives, and they may die before us. All of these possibilities will bring our own sense of helplessness to the fore, making us feel out of control. At times, we may feel like we are complete failures.

The sooner we accept that we cannot control our children's experiences and how they feel about them, the sooner we can release our unrealistic fantasies that our children should have only happy feelings. Our children are sovereign beings who are entitled to experience life any way they desire. If they desire to be sad at the beach, that is their choice. Who are we to tell them how to feel? I still remember the photographer at my daughter's two-year birthday party telling me, "I tried hard to get her to smile but, boy, it was really difficult." I remember immediately feeling as if there was something wrong with her or me. Why couldn't she just smile and be happy like the other kids? It was only upon later reflection that I saw how we parents are often like the happiness police, shouting out commands to our children: "Smile! Be Happy! Don't Cry!" In giving these orders, we tell them to ignore their authentic feelings and just feel what we want them to feel so that we can feel good about ourselves.

Our children are not our puppets or our canvas upon which to paint our desires and expectations. They are their own beings with their own needs and temperaments. If they choose to be in a sulky mood at a really fun amusement park, that is their right. They own their feelings. As long as they don't harm anyone else, our kids, and every human, have a right to their own feelings. When we release ourselves and others from the need for them to be happy, we communicate an intrinsic acceptance with life. We realize that wanting only happy life experiences is an infantile way to live.

Life is not biased toward any one feeling. Life just is. Sometimes it's this way and sometimes it's that way. It doesn't dictate how we feel about it. That is up to us. Rain can make someone happy, while it makes someone else miserable. Rain just is. It doesn't mean to create a reaction in us. The reaction is all on us. In our unconsciousness, we believe that our reactions are ruled by life. As we awaken, we realize our reactions have nothing to do with the external world and all to do with our inner self.

What if we replaced the notion of happiness with something more lasting and attainable? What if we replaced it with presence? Presence implies an embrace of *all* our experiences, the ones that cause happiness *and* the ones that cause pain. When we approach life with the awareness that happiness and sadness are an inextricable part of life, we stop judging life as "good" or "bad." Life just is. Being open to its teachings, no matter what emotions they create within us, is to be in presence. Presence is an everlasting quality we cultivate when we accept life however it shows up, in all its wide array of possibilities. When we surrender to life, we allow ourselves and our children to go through its peaks and valleys with equanimity and joy. We don't judge life according to how it makes us feel but instead accept it for the teachings it bestows. This perspective allows us to release our anxieties around our own and our children's experiences. In this way, we set ourselves and them free to engage in life's as-is without trepidation or resistance.

Let's now deconstruct what success means. When we talk about success, we mean high accolades, high achievement, high status, and a high bank account. This is how culture has defined success and how most of us see it. That's why we plan our children's entire childhood to meet those standards. The ability of our children to compete for the most prestigious universities and sports teams becomes every parent's focus. When our children can't check these boxes, we see them, and ourselves, as failures. As a result, we live with high stress and anxiety in an attempt to ward off the possibility of this potential doom.

When we begin to allow our children to experience worth based

on their intrinsic sense of well-being, and not on extrinsic culturally prescribed standards, we endorse our *being* state rather than
our doing state. Our being begins to matter more than what we do.
After all, we are human beings, not human doings.

Awakening means we *un*subscribe from culture's definition of
success and create new paths of authentic self-discovery where we
set our own markers for achievement and progress. As we do so, we
realize we are fully worthy as we are, without craving what culture
told us will fill us up.

When we mother our children from a place of wholeness, we cannot help but project this sense of completeness onto them. We stop
seeing them as lesser-than, incomplete, or broken. We see them as
perfect just as they are, in all their imperfections. We don't see their
C grades as meaning anything less about who they are. We don't
impose culture's standards of achievement on them but instead
allow them to blossom at their own pace and according to their
standards.

Culture says life is a competition and a struggle. While we understand that life can be tough sometimes, we don't subscribe to
this scarcity model of life. As we grow in inner abundance, we
allow our kids to grow in abundance as well. We teach them that
there are infinite ways to live life, and their path is as valid as anyone else's.

Our children are not meant to be "mini-mes," nor are they our
puppets or trophies. They are here to grow into the unique spirits
they already are, and to manifest their destiny in the manner that
works most authentically for them.

Redefining Motherhood

When we begin to see our children as teachers for our own inner
growth, motherhood undergoes a drastic overhaul. Unless we heal
our own childhood wounds, we will project our inner "holes" onto
our children. Through acknowledging this, we can use the mother-

hood journey as a portal to our evolution. Motherhood becomes less about our children's happiness and success and more about our inner healing. We go beyond the role of mother and shed the ego this comes with and instead enter something deeper—our mothering essence. Now motherhood is no longer about the children we produce or create and more about the inauthenticities we shed and release.

Looking within means to ask ourselves, Where does this need to be omnipotent in our children's lives come from? and, Why is it that I need my child to be happy and successful? Both answers will reveal our desperate sense of inner helplessness and unworthiness. We come to see that we have been projecting our inner lack onto our children. When we do this, we then seek to correct, fix, and mend this inner lack in them, little realizing that they aren't lacking at all. All the lack is coming from within us. Until we can see how we do this to our children as well as our other intimate relationships, we will keep parasitically drawing from the other's worth, hoping a few droplets will salve our inner wounds.

Awakening involves shattering the cultural archetypes of happiness and success. When we realize that it isn't our job to create happiness or success within our kids, we not only set our kids free, we free ourselves also.

Releasing our enmeshment with our children is one of the hardest spiritual tasks of any mother. This means we glean a sense of worth from our own being, separate from that of our kids. We do our own inner work and absolve our kids from the burden of carrying the weight of our expectations. Our purpose shifts from wanting the best for our kids so that we feel good about ourselves to wanting the best for ourselves so that we don't use our kids to feel worthy.

When we shift our purpose as mothers from an egoic and unconscious parenting style to a more evolved and conscious one, we move from thinking of ourselves as our children's leaders and commanders to being their guides and chaperones. We realize our highest purpose is to see them as our teachers, our awakeners, and learn from the lessons they teach us. We are to move from our place in front of the line to walking by their side, if they let us, or behind them if they don't. We now see ourselves as conduits, ushers, and fellow travelers with our children on this journey called life.

When we mothers forget our true nature and are distracted by culture's cacophony, we betray our spiritual core. Culture tells us to be anxious and controlling, craving and striving. We believe this is how we need to be, so we get impatient and frustrated, strident and demanding. Our children feel this and bolt.

When we beat our children, scream at them, or shame them in some way, we are going against our true nature. This is not who we are, though it may be who we were taught to be, first toward ourselves and then toward our children. The result is that our children lose their connection to their authentic self and buy into a toxic and dysfunctional way of being.

We need to shift the paradigm on motherhood. Our purpose as a mother is to raise our kids to adulthood healthily, period. When we focus on this, we are warm, nurturing, and nonstressed. Culture polluted our authentic purpose and added all sorts of artificial ingredients into it, such as making sure kids are happy, skinny, popular, and successful. When we fall prey to these additional cultural dictates, we come out of our natural motherly element and go against our heart. Now we are anxious, irritable, rageful, and resentful.

When we let go of culture's dogma and dictates, we once again enter into the heart and soul of motherhood, which is to nurture and support our kids to independence. The future needs us mothers to resist culture's abduction of who we truly are. When we do, we not only free ourselves to be authentic, but we allow this in our children. There is simply no power greater to change the world than a mother's.

17

The Lies About Beauty and Youth

We believe that our youth should be preserved like jam in a jar
Our skin should stay smooth like whipped cream
Our bodies forever flexible like an acrobatic wonder
Our hair shiny like the finest draped silk
Clinging to the beauty standard, we stop living in beauty.

I don't think I have known a woman who has consistently declared, "I am really happy with how I look and wouldn't change a thing about my appearance." Isn't that telling? Almost tragic? It's so common to be down on ourselves for our looks that we don't even question the ubiquity of it. While I am sure there are men who are not completely happy with their looks, it's not something they typically moan about. But women? It's standard practice.

External pressures show up in all sorts of ways, but none so severe for women as those from the beauty industry. Whether we directly succumb to it or not, we are all mired in it to one degree or another. Culture has made us base our worth on the flawlessness of our complexion, the size 0 of our body, and our eternal youth. Caught in a toxic pattern of endlessly competing with other women, we are stuck in the lair of comparing ourselves to them. At the gym, when we see other women working out, at the grocery store as we thumb through magazines, and at the movies as we watch the actresses light up the screen, we continually ask ourselves, How does my body measure up compared to her breasts, her nose, her smile, her legs, her buttocks, her eyes?

Whether we are blatant about it or silently merciless, most of us are hard on ourselves when it comes to how we look. When we look in the mirror, we notice all our flaws before we notice our beauty—the bulge in our stomach, the wrinkles, the stretch marks, or the cellulite. Our inner critic is relentless.

Slaves to the Mirror

For as long as I can remember, every day when I awakened, I looked in the mirror and found fault with my face and body. My eyes zeroed in on my wrinkles and cellulite. This was all I saw—wrinkles and cellulite. The only difference in the new me versus the old me is that now I manage, on most days, not to spiral into a vicious self-attack and can stay above the water in terms of derision and scorn.

In the past, I entered a relentless inner critical dialogue about how I would simply never be good enough. My mind would obsess over all the things about my face and body that were wrong—all the things culture has said are wrong, such as my wavy and *not* straight hair, my darker or rather browner and *not* white color, my curvy and *not* skinny body, my cellulite-heavy and *not* smooth skin, my rubbing and *not*-gapped inner thighs, my short and *not* long legs.

I loathed myself to such a degree that I worked myself into an eating disorder. Do you know where I first learned about bulimia? From my best friend. We were barely sixteen years old. And who did she learn it from? From another group of young teenage girls who had been bulimic for a while. It was as if all these young women knew something I didn't. They had a casual attitude about it all to the tune of, "Oh, I just eat what I want and then I throw up and don't put on weight." I was astounded. I had never heard of such a thing. I thought to myself, "Wow, I might as well try it."

Thankfully for me, I was never good at the technique nor did I feel good about the whole process. I felt averse to it both physically and psychologically. I knew something was wrong with this idea and that it couldn't possibly be healthy to be hurting my body in this callous way. I finally stopped after a few months but not because I had entered a wholesome self-acceptance. I just didn't like the process of eating and throwing my food back up. I wish I had stopped because of my growing self-love. I can honestly say that if there was another more pleasurable process of extricating the food from my body, I would have grabbed it.

Why do eating disorders predominate in women compared to men? The reason is, we are first gauged on our external beauty and only secondarily on our inner qualities. So objectified are we that we internalize this oppression and soon become our own biggest objectifiers and oppressors. Before we know it, we act as if our body is on display at a museum. We critique our body in pieces—the ear lobe, the inner thigh, the lack of triceps, the fat ankles. We then want to have the best of every feature possible—the best lips, eye lashes, cheek bones, and jaw line. We take apart our face and no longer see it as a whole. We forget that we are a composite, to be appreciated in our totality. Do you know how toxic this is for our well-being?

It was only in my thirties, after birthing my daughter, that I realized something had to change within me or I would pass on this internal tyranny to her. Unless I learned to accept and celebrate my body just as it was, I would surely send the message that a woman's worth is tied to her looks. I began to do some serious inner work by deconstructing every flawed belief system around how I looked and what culture said about it.

It took a while. I began to realize that it wasn't my body that was flawed, but culture's way of perceiving a woman's body. I had taken in culture's distorted perspective and turned it on myself. There is no such thing as a flawed body, only a healthy body or an unhealthy body. Once I realized this, I began to release culture's indoctrination. Although I still suffer from intermittent internal tyranny, I have come to a place where I can now more deeply accept the body and face I was born with.

No matter what culture says, the fact that we buy into it and perpetuate our own vilification is a sign that we have, on a subconscious level, accepted what culture says. This is a hard pill to swallow. We endorse what culture decides is beautiful. In doing so, we vacate our own unique worth and genetic lineage.

For generations women the world over have betrayed themselves more than culture ever has. We sell ourselves as unimportant, insignificant, and irrelevant. And do you know to whom we sell ourselves? To a phantom "other," meaning everyone "out there." To the cosmetic and plastic surgery industry, to fashion labels, to culture, the media, the patriarchy, and to the highest bidder. They begin to own us more than we own ourselves. My goal is not for us to annihilate our submission to culture completely. We may still choose to wax our upper lip, shave our underarms, and shape our eyebrows. The point of this exposé is for us to make as many conscious choices as we can so that we don't robotically fall into culture's ways without discernment.

The Colonization of Beauty

There is a standard of beauty that has colonized the world at large. It hyper-focuses on white skin, young skinny bodies, light eyes, and blonde hair. The preferred shape of the body has gone through many iterations over time, some decades preferring flat-chested bony bodies, with other decades showing proclivities for buxom and curvy bodies. Regardless, the skin needs to be white. The whiter the better—and the younger the better. This standard of beauty has plagued women, young and old, crucifying us with its unrelenting parameters.

When the term *all-American beauty* is used, it is typically associated with a thin, blonde, young, blue-eyed, white woman. The Miss America pageant didn't even allow women of color to enter until the 1940s. Until then, the contestants needed to be of "good health and of the white race." Even today most magazine covers and billboards showcase the white face, blonde hair, and the white body. A young girl of color will need to forage the covers to find her own type reflected back at her.

Most black women and other women of color will attest to growing up with a gnawing feeling of never being beautiful enough. From flat-ironing their hair, bleaching their skin, or tying their bodies in tight-fitting shapewear, women have been begging to fit into this white standard of beauty. For black and brown women to realize that "black is beautiful" and "brown is beautiful" has been slow coming.

Our current standards of beauty belie the underlying preponderance of cultural racism and agism. By stratifying the concept of beauty to the rigid and narrow definitions it has, our current culture has tortured the self-esteem of millions of girls around the globe. As women, it's our responsibility to challenge the current status quo around beauty, redefining what it means for each of us. This is the only way to embrace an expanded consciousness about our worth, one that divorces itself from the current beauty paradigm.

Nature gave us our time for youthful beauty but never intended us to hold on to it forever. Look at the whole of nature—everything ages and dies. There is no struggle involved. So where did we learn that we need to fight nature and resist the passing of time? From culture, that's where. We were hypnotized to believe in something that nature didn't intend for us.

The ravages of time are going to wrinkle our forehead and sag our chin, and there is nothing we can do about it. Culture tells us that aging is an anathema and to be avoided at all costs. So now a woman experiences a huge inner split, which she then seeks to resolve through artificial means. It may not be her preference to desire fillers or Botox, yet she finds herself buckling under a cacophonous inner critic that she has inherited from culture, relentlessly punishing herself for going through the normal passages of time.

Men do not tie their sense of worth to how they look like women do. This is rampantly clear. Each time I get on stage in a lineup of speakers, I am abundantly aware of how women fall prey to different standards of beauty. The men typically go on stage in plain clothes and regular shoes, without much ado about anything. But the women? There are makeup artists, hair stylists, and uncomfortable high heels. Of course, not all women obsess about their appearance, but it is safe to assume that most do. This is how culture has indoctrinated us. Because of this, we tie our intrinsic sense of worth to our external appearance. In doing this we suffer greatly.

By undermining the beauty we were born with, downgrading it, snubbing it, and making excuses for it, we give our power away each and every day to the "whitified" patriarchy. By subscribing to the standard, subjugating our bodies to endure hours of daily torture, we decimate our worth and entertain a lesser-than-ness that isn't ours to own. We constantly try to mask, adorn, embellish, and disguise our natural beauty. We wear only black, for example, or big baggy clothes. We use special makeup and lighting, or we color our hair and subject it to all sorts of chemical processes, spending thousands of dollars on shoes and clothes with fancy labels, or wearing all sorts of fake hair, lashes, fillers, and implants to hide who we are. It's our way of pretending that who we are in the natural shouldn't be the way it is.

How do we begin to create a new standard of beauty for ourselves? We start by understanding what we are up against. Once we do, we consciously embrace our own body in all its ages, shapes, and forms. As we enter into a deeper union with ourselves, we are conscious to educate our daughters, the younger generations, to embrace themselves. We teach them about how culture may or may not accept their appearance, and how they can combat its psychological effects. By bringing this issue to light through conscious dialogue, we can help young girls create a better body awareness and self-image.

Moving Beyond Beautiful

What I am about to say now is a huge paradigm shift in what is considered politically correct. The popular notion among new age feminists is to call ourselves beautiful and find every piece of us stunning. "Beautiful" is not just an adjective. It implies a judgment of "goodness." There are some descriptions that go beyond mere qualifiers into the realm of good-versus-bad. *Beautiful* is one of those terms, like *pretty* or *ugly*.

I began to shift my internal paradigm when I moved away from my desire to call things beautiful and instead started to call things as they are. If one part of my body is flabby, I am going to call it flabby. I don't need to judge it as good or bad. It's just *flabby*. What is the big deal about flabby? If another part of my body is chubby, I am going to call it chubby. There's nothing good or bad about it. It's just *chubby*. If I have crow's feet around my eyes, that's just the way it is.

I don't need to say, "I have crow's feet *and* they are beautiful." Needing to say this implies a measure of insecurity. True acceptance of our bodies would allow our bodies to be noticed as they are, without the labels of good or bad. Because we are so against the words *fat*, *cellulite*, and *wrinkles*, we hear these words as an insult. This is a cultural projection. What if they just *are*?

When we hear our daughters or women in general say, "I'm so fat," our instinct is to say, "No you're not, you're so thin. I wish I was thin like you." Or if they were to say, "I hate how ugly I am," we would immediately pipe in, "You're not ugly, you're beautiful. Look at your lovely smile and your cute, perky nose." Without realizing, we engage in adulating our children, our girls especially, in our efforts to lend them a sense of belonging, perhaps the one we never had. Little do we realize that we are in fact perpetuating their unworthiness.

When we compliment children about their looks and dismiss their sense of loathing, we unwittingly endorse their insecurities and magnify them. So what should we do? The solution isn't to change the game, it's to stop playing the game. When a daughter or young woman says she is fat, we don't refute her because to do so is to engage in a false dialogue. Instead we can say something like, "You are who you are. Don't label it. Don't judge it. Accept yourself as you are and love yourself for that. Instead of looking at yourself with loathing, look at yourself with appreciation. Love whatever it is you are judging. Remove the comparisons and the negativity. Instead, celebrate that this is how your body protects you, this is how your shape endows you, and this is how your face reflects you. Don't try to be someone else. Be you. For this to happen, you need to accept every part of yourself. Once you accept yourself as you are, you can then choose to change something if it feels authentic to you."

I still remember when my daughter commented on the ways in which the flesh on my underarms swung left to right. She was delighted by this. "Mommy make your helicopter wings fly," she would say. My instinct was to hide them or to tell her they were beautiful or strong. After pausing a moment, I realized that I didn't have to say anything. I could just show her my embrace of my body through acceptance. No need for labels, adjectives, dialogue, re-sistance, or affirmations of beauty or strength. If I truly accepted myself as-is, what was there to resist, protest, or argue about? Each time she would want to see my "helicopter wings," I laughed in de-light and began flying around the room ensuring that the fat jig-gled all over. She would literally keel over in delight. I would also remind her that her arms may not have so much jiggle and that she shouldn't feel bad that she couldn't fly because everyone's body is different, with different powers.

Just as words can heal, they can shame. Ultimately the words we say to ourselves are the only ones that matter. There will always be those on the outside who use words to shame us. When this hap-pens, although it's difficult, we need to step back and realize that they do so out of their own insecurity. Having said this, sometimes if someone says we are fat, we need to pause before reacting as if it were a shaming pejorative. What if we are just this fat? For exam-ple, if someone told me that I have cellulite on my thighs, would I consider it shaming or the truth? The fact is I do have cellulite. So now what? Do I get upset by this fact and feel ashamed? Or do I see it as a neutral fact and move on? Do you see my point? Culture makes us feel bad about cellulite or our fat as if it's a bad thing to have, when in fact it's perfectly natural. Culture does this with almost every part of our body that doesn't fit the westernized, whiti-fied standard of beauty.

Most often, words are just pointers. When they are used to shame another, they move from mere communication tools to weapons of emotional destruction. Take the word *obese*. It's a reference to a med-ical disease of having a BMI over a certain index. It's a health-related issue, not a moral pejorative. However, if one were to call another obese, it could be seen as fat-shaming, as opposed to being used as a medical descriptor. Of course, many use these terms to slander and defame. There will always be those who do this to gain egoic domi-nance. Again, the power to react to these words lies within us. When we internalize shame, we have, in effect, given our authority away.

The point is not what others say but what we internalize. When we are unable to fully accept our imperfect body, we cannot expect that others will. This doesn't mean that we don't exercise our bod-ies or curl our hair for a party, or even inject Botox, if that is what we choose. It means that we first arrive at a place of an honest ac-knowledgment of our ego and then make choices accordingly. We discern, weigh, and balance, instead of robotically falling prey to culture or our insecurity.

When we move away from how culture has set us up, we begin to stop seeing the imperfections and stop calling our body parts "flawed." And if we do, we immediately question: According to what? We realize that our judgments are faulty, stemming from false archetypes. So if the archetypes are themselves false, then the judgments have to be false as well. It's quite possible, then, that there is no problem with our body parts at all. Through this con-stant questioning of what we have automatically indoctrinated, we move away from objectification into wholeness.

The Cocreation of Objectification

What I am about to say will trigger a few of you. Why? I am asking women to take some responsibility for their misery. This is never a comfortable thing to do, yet only when we take ownership of the ways in which we participate in our reality, knowingly or unknowingly, will we empower ourselves, our sisters, and our daughters.

Ask any couple which of them buys the most clothes, more beauty products, and takes a longer time to get ready for major events, and it will most likely be the woman. One of the first things we ask ourselves when preparing for an event is, What am I going to wear? What shoes will I wear with my outfit?

Ask any woman why she dresses up the way she does, and she will promptly say, "Because it makes me feel good! I dress up for myself!" And while this is true, it is not the whole truth. The other part of the truth is something we don't prefer to readily admit. And the other part is this: we highly covet being desired. It is as much a part of our wiring as it is part of a male's to hunt and desire. Even though we say we don't, we seek this desire and subconsciously tailor much of our existence around it. We can pretend we like to adorn, embellish, and disguise ourselves because it makes us happy, but we wouldn't be telling the whole truth.

How do I know this to be true? I look at how we are when we are on our own. No makeup, no accessories, braless boobs, same old T-shirt, dirty sweat pants. So if we are okay being like this on our own but then dress to the nines when we go outside, it's illogical to say we aren't doing this largely for others. Not even our partners get the treatment strangers do.

Every time I challenge my girlfriends and say, "You just love getting compliments, don't you?" they refuse to own up to it. They inevitably retort, "I do not! I do this for myself." It's hard for us to own that we may have a subconscious agenda for getting dolled up. In truth, there is nothing to be ashamed of. In fact, as I said, it is part of our wiring to want to feel desired. So why not admit it? Why be ashamed of it?

In fact, I would go so far as to say that another subconscious agenda we have is using our beauty to our advantage. We curve our bodies in a particular way in photos, taking "our best side." We put one leg in front of another when we stand so that we give the appearance of a longer leg. We touch our face up with powder, use perfume, and volumize our hair. We make sure to take a few minutes longer on our appearance for an interview. We subconsciously know that we have this "thing" called beauty on our side, and we certainly try our best to play to it. Again, we don't like to admit these things, partly because it's a double-edged sword for us. Part of us "uses" our beauty and another part of us abhors the fact that we feel the need to do so.

This is the first place where our co-participation in culture's objectification starts. While we feel burdened by it, we have bought into it in our own way. Unless we can own this buying in, we will not rise above it in a conscious way and nothing will really change.

Ultimately the truth is that no one can tell us to look a certain way or tell us how to feel about how we look. This is fully up to us. Each time we look in the mirror and critique ourselves because we don't match a certain standard, we are cocreating our own objectification and subjugation. We could well look in the mirror and say, "I don't give a damn about how others see me or how I look right now. I am who I am and I look how I look, and that's it!"

Imagine the psychological repercussions that would ensue if we adopted such a stance. For one, we would feel an immediate dissolution of all the pressures and anxieties we have been harboring with our desire to fit in. We would immediately let go of all of the mental plague we typically go through when we get ready for an event or when we believe we don't look a particular way. Not only would our anxiety fade, our self-esteem would rocket. This daring embrace of who we are renders the opinion of culture and others irrelevant.

When a woman's first white hairs sprout, she rushes to color them lest she be considered old. When a man turns gray, he is considered distinguished and worldly. If a woman has a paunch, she is considered unattractive, yet few blink an eye when a man has one. If she balds, a woman will rush to cover the balding spots with a wig or a scarf. If he turns bald, it's considered normal. If she goes to a party drably dressed, she will be judged tenfold. If he does the same, he is blown off as "just being a guy." Women have our own code and men have theirs.

We don't care as much if our sons look scruffy or eat extra butter on their toast, but we are not as nonchalant with our girls. We want them to watch their weight and pay attention to how their hair and skin look. In subtle and not-so-subtle ways, we pass on the same standards we were stifled by to our girls. The standards for men and women are vastly different.

The first price we pay arises out of our denial. Claiming that we strive for all this extra beautification "because it makes us happy" is denial. The beautification doesn't make us happy. The compliments or the feeling we get when others appreciate us does. Big difference. If we owned that we like compliments and attention, we would do ourselves a favor. We would see how we choose to succumb to this need versus pretending it didn't exist.

Ownership brings empowerment. What is wrong with saying, "I love compliments. I love being told I am beautiful. I love for others to see my body and comment on it." Do you see what I mean? We enact a double standard. We dress to the hilt but then complain about all the attention we get. Also, let's remember, if the attention was from some gorgeous Hollywood-type stranger, we wouldn't mind as much as if it was a regular stranger on the road. We are filled with ambiguity around this.

The second price we pay arises out of our own participation in raising the beauty bar. When we submit to insane standards of beauty by stuffing our bodies with implants or "enhancing" our image beyond recognition, we are complicit in the disempowerment of women. By constantly seeking "the next best thing" in beauty, we endorse the idea that there is something more to fix and improve, sending this message to other women. Without consciously realizing it, by constantly tweaking and fixing our bodies to conform to the standard, we keep raising the beauty bar.

Falling prey to the latest trends keeps us feeling like we can never keep up. Again, we need to be aware that *we* are falling prey. No one is necessarily making us do so. In "keeping up with the Kardashians," we make those around us feel as if they too should keep up. You know how it is. If three out of ten women dress up, the seven who didn't end up feeling uncomfortable because they look like they just rolled out of bed. When three have butt implants, they now make the other seven with regular butts look exactly that—regular. Suddenly, what was once considered "regular," is now considered something to be ashamed of.

When we wear fake lashes, we make a statement, raise the beauty bar, and influence the beauty culture around us. When we wear red lipstick, we do so as well. Same with a push-up bra, and the use of flattering filters in our social media photos. In these seemingly innocuous ways, we participate in what culture has said is attractive, yet we can now realize that these are not innocuous choices at all. They are anything but. They are lethal choices we make that then cocreate the beauty culture that we bemoan daily.

Take the simple act of wearing hair extensions and wigs. We wear them to give others the impression that our hair is more lustrous, silkier, or more coiffed than it actually is. We like the compliments we receive. We feel better about ourselves. If only things ended there. We now set the bar for hair higher than it would have been had women just been using their regular hair. There is a cascading domino effect from this one act. Another woman looks at the one wearing hair extensions and may covet the look. She notices how this woman garners attention and praise. She desires that for herself. The next thing she knows, she is scouring the internet for a similar weave. The sad thing is that she used to be just fine with her hair. She accepted it for what it was. But seeing how other women manipulate their hair and how this gets them positive attention, she now suddenly feels insecure about her hair.

This all may be happening at a subconscious level, but it is how women unwittingly set the stage for their misery. Little do we realize that by constantly striving to look better, and feeling insecure and unworthy, we actually patronize the patriarchy that defines us. This is why it's so pivotal for us to awaken to our own subjugation and objectification.

Self-acceptance is what it's all about, at the end of the day. When we are able to enter this state for ourselves, we don't degrade other women or exalt them. We simply appreciate the beauty in each of us—all forms and ages. We recognize our diversity and allow ourselves to differ from the norms culture places on us. When we feel "good enough," we stop striving and craving to be better than the best. Emotional liberation arrives when we free ourselves from the clutches of being defined by anyone outside of ourselves. This could not be truer than in the case of defining beauty according to our own standard and vision.

18

The Lies About Niceness

Be nice, be polite, be kind
Be sweet, be quiet, don't be angry
Trained to be mute, we learn to girdle up
Straightjacketed into compliance
We allow our power to be heisted.

It's really simple, Mom. It's one word, two letters. N. O." My daughter, Maia, was giving me a quick tutorial on how to say no. She said to me, "Mom, you know what you are? A really thick, plush carpet that everyone loves to walk on!" Out of the mouths of babes indeed. She was right. If there was one core issue of mine, my greatest Achilles' heel, it was my inability to say no.

Do you know why it's so hard for me to say no? Simple. I was raised to say yes. I was raised to be "nice," and nice girls said yes a lot. They said yes even when they really wanted to say no. They said yes because they were trained to care about other people's feelings more than their own. After all, kind girls are nice to everyone. They don't cause an uproar, commotion, or drama. They are easygoing and simple.

I know I was not raised in an unusual way. I know there are millions of women who were raised to be little toy soldiers in their parents' army. Good soldiers follow instructions, don't ask too many questions, certainly don't protest too loudly, and readily comply.

The more we do this, the more others are happy with us and we receive the validation we were trained to desperately crave.

If there has been one curse women have suffered, it's the curse of niceness. Boys can be boys, as in loud, boisterous, and noisy. But girls? They must be nice. What this means is simply that we please those around us, allowing them to get their way. We are supposed to take care of others' feelings at all costs.

Think about this mandate for a minute. On the one hand, taking care of others' feelings is a basic ingredient in the daily comings and goings of a relationship. We don't want to be outright nasty and rude. But, on the other hand, this is an impossible mandate. Can we ever really take care of another's feelings? It's literally only possible if we are willing to completely kill any individuality within us and bend, twist, circle, and spiral into any shape, size, and form in order to make them happy. This is soul suicide at its finest.

Do you know how much time women have wasted on trying to fit into the role of the "nice" girl? To get them to like us and call us "sweet" and "polite"? How many times have we wanted to say no, but the word stays stuck deep in our belly? How many times have we avoided conflict out of a paralytic fear of confrontation? How many raises have we never asked our bosses for? How many sexual advances have we not protected ourselves against? Or how many dysfunctional relationships have we not walked out of, all because we were trying to be "nice"?

Take the husband who wants his wife to have sex with him in a particular way or with a particular frequency. If she refuses, he gets upset. Does that mean she is not nice? Or consider the mother who wants her daughter to call her every day or she gets hurt. When the daughter fails to do so, does this mean she doesn't care about her mom? Then there's the friend who wants you to only be with her at a party or else she feels insecure.

Where is the line between being nice to another and being authentic? How can we take care of another's feelings without betraying ourselves? How can we be true to our own feelings and boundaries while also taking care of another?

These are the pivotal questions we need to ask if we are to awaken to our true self, which longs for the freedom to be authentic. In order for this freedom to be granted, we need to step away from the mandate to "be nice" and move into a new declaration of who we truly are, guided by the imperative to be authentic.

When Femininity Turns Toxic

Shushed into being nice and conciliatory, every girl receives the message that her will, autonomy, and voice are not as important as that of others. She learns to yield, comply, and mold herself into all sorts of shapes depending on what others need. Constantly capitulating to others, she soon all but forgets she even exists.

When Mandy came to me for a session, she was 120 pounds overweight. Beneath her layers was a stunning woman. Mandy described herself as "the classic codependent empath." It was as if codependency was an addiction she had no control over, not a choice she made on a daily basis. She had been married to the same man for over thirty years even though she knew he repeatedly cheated on her. She reported feeling listless and passionless in the marriage, yet she chose to stay. "I don't know why I stay," she admitted, "I just do." Emotionally paralyzed, she said she was unable to leave. Her role in the family was to caretake those around her and serve their needs. To leave her husband felt sacrilegious to her.

Despite her weight, Mandy was a person who was invisible to herself. She joked, "I know I don't look invisible, but I am." In her desire to be a loving wife and mother, she had completely sacrificed her identity. She looked at me in bewilderment when I explained to her how she had developed a toxic femininity. We have all been hearing about toxic masculinity, but toxic femininity?

When a woman is firmly rooted in the feminine dimension, she is in touch with her feelings and capacity for openness. She is able to receive and nurture, connecting and communing with ease and grace. She is infinitely flexible, cooperative, a communicator, and tribe builder. She is as at home with the young as with the old, with the weak as with the strong. The feminine principle is life-giving and life-affirming. It vibrates with an awakened energy of interdependence and a reverential tolerance for diversity. It's our natural way, our giving way.

So what is toxic femininity? It's the feminine principle at its most extreme form. It typically begins when a young girl is raised in a highly unconscious childhood where she instinctively learns that being silent is a smart survival strategy. This is a typical occurrence when the young girl grows up in the following ways:

She has parents who are controlling and helicoptering.
She has parents who are suffering from their own traumas.
She has parents who are neglectful and/or aggressively
    threatening.

In this case, the parents are more concerned about themselves than the young girl's self-expression. There isn't enough emotional space for her to fly free.

Children need homes to be infinitely flexible for their unique temperament to blossom. When the home is filled with the unconsciousness of an older generation, the children are manipulated into fitting into the system. Instead of the system morphing itself to accommodate the unique needs of the children, it demands that the children give up who they are in order to fit into the existing system. When parents are wrapped up in their own attachments, either to their own belief systems or to their past childhood wounds, children are made to feel as if they are part of the woodwork. They fade in to fit in, otherwise the house will fall down.

Children, especially sensitive girls, sense the emotional fragility of their parents and home. They immediately jump to the rescue and do their part to glue things together as best they can. Instead of using their energy to develop their own mind and beliefs, they expend all their resources on trying to manage an unmanageable situation.

A girl growing up in such a home detects early on how fragile everyone is and realizes that her voice, her feelings, and her fears will break the proverbial camel's back. So what does she do? She squelches her feelings. Instead of tuning into herself, she becomes a master at reading other people's energy. Her survival is based on her ability to read others. In this way, her entire focus is on conflict avoidance and allowing others to supersede her will. She all but physically dies. So passive and dependent does she become that she stops exercising her free spirit. So afraid is she to use her own direction and power that she stays infantile and regressed. The powerful qualities of the feminine mutate into an extreme version and end up as a perversion. This is how toxic femininity harnesses the original template of the woman and ruptures it till it looks nothing like what it was meant to.

When I traced Mandy's current situation to her childhood, the trauma bonds became more apparent. Mandy lost her two older siblings and mother to a house fire. She was at kindergarten when it happened. After that, she lived with her father who became a rageful alcoholic. She had many surrogate mothers who came in and out of her life, but no one to really turn to with her grief. Starting in first grade, most nights she watched her father pass out drunk. She remembers waking herself up for school and handling her homework all by herself. Mandy learned early that there was no room for her to exist. Psychologically, she thought of herself as having died with her sisters and mother in the fire. Today she was just a breathing relic of what befell them.

Mandy grew up to be an addictive eater. She was obese by the age of seven and had never been able to lose the weight. "I use food to stuff my feelings down," she admitted. "The act of chewing soothes me. It's my only comfort. I guess as a child there was no one to help me with my feelings, so food and TV was all I had. I haven't stopped chewing or numbing myself with TV since then."

Mandy had all but lost herself. But if we asked her family or friends about her trauma, I bet they wouldn't even know this part of her. They would be shocked, actually. They might say something

like, "But she is always so happy and easygoing. She never gets upset or angry."

This is what the classic "nice" girl does. So disconnected is she
from her authentic inner voice that she simply goes along with
whatever others tell her to do. This is much easier to do than the inner work required to become whole. The nicer she is, the more she
receives validation and accolades. This, in turn, further validates
her silence.

Our original template of nurturing love gets destroyed completely and in its place is a toxic replacement. Here are some of the
ways this happens:

Adaptability mutates into inauthenticity.
Cooperation mutates into servility.
Sensitivity mutates into fragility.
Connectivity mutates into dependency.
Patience mutates into paralysis.
Harmonizing mutates into conflict aversion.

Toxic femininity has the power to all but annihilate the self. It
has such an influence over our authentic soul that it leaves us in a
complete fog. It has been so long since we felt our power that we
don't even remember our true selves. When we realize we have
traded being authentic for being nice, we are at first disoriented.
For so long, we have only known how to be one way–nice. Understanding how the need to be nice has undermined our authenticity
is a shock.

As Mandy began to awaken, she saw how her being nice was not
only avoiding conflict in her life but also avoiding transparency
within her own being. She was, in effect, living a lie. This is what
happens when we pivot our lives to focus on external relationships.
By catering to others' moods and needs constantly, we stop paying
attention to our own. This way, we avoid the struggle that comes
with figuring out what our authentic feelings are. By bypassing this inner struggle, we think we are at peace and in balance.

This couldn't be further from the truth. We are actually way out of whack. This is why "nice" girls often have addiction issues. Although typically to food, this addiction could be to any of a range of substances, from alcohol to opioids, to prescription pain killers, to workaholism—basically anything that allows her to suppress her inner voice and squelch her truth. The only way to compensate for this utter denial of our authentic voice is to over-rely on something else. We create a false, and often lethal, proxy system, one that eventually devours every last shard of who we are.

In order for women infected with the curse of niceness to wake up, they need to infuse their psyches with a newfound force. In order to jolt themselves into active empowerment, they need to inject healthy doses of masculinity. Only when they are able to balance out their psyches with masculine energy will they transcend their current suffering.

The Power of Masculinity

When we live inauthentically, we are in false relationships with the world. How can we not be? If we lie to ourselves, we lie to others. Therefore the persona that others see as ourselves is an illusion. Just as we don't know who we are, others don't know us either. They are in a relationship with someone who doesn't even exist—a relationship with our ego. If we are in our ego and a state of inauthenticity when dealing with others, then they are too. This is how one person's lack of consciousness keeps others mired in the same fear and dishonesty. Entering true intimacy requires, before all else, an honest and true intimacy with ourselves.

When we deny our voice, we actually allow others, men in particular, to behave rather poorly. We train the others in our lives—our partners and our kids—to be insensitive to our needs and desires. Little do we realize that by *not* speaking up for ourselves, we are actually not protecting anyone's soul, just their ego. More than this, we are protecting our own past patterns of servility.

When we women "take care" of the others in our lives and trample their own ability to rise up to the challenge of becoming better humans, we are not being loving *at all*. You read that right. *We are not loving at all*. In fact, we are downright selfish. We are thieves, robbing the other of the right to confront that truth as it needs to be. We don't respect the other's potential when we kowtow to their every need. By treating them as if they cannot handle our authentic truth, or handle the end of their dependency on us, we actually communicate our disrespect for them. We don't believe they can cope with these realities. By not challenging them to cope, we keep them infantile and stuck.

Ask any woman if they have struggled with creating boundaries. I guarantee most will say yes. Saying no doesn't come easy to most of us, especially if it means conflict and dissension. Most of us are nauseated by conflict. It can literally make us physically ill, so terrified are we. The trauma of growing up with unconscious parents who couldn't regulate or process their own big feelings left such an inner scar on us that we now bolt at the slightest echo of emotional intensity.

We are conditioned to avoid any sort of conflict because we associate it with anger. Anger and other intense emotions scarred us so much as children that we learned to avoid them at all costs. To be around anger, our own or another's, is often downright paralyzing because it goes against the grain of "niceness." We have been trained to avoid anger at all costs by pleasing the other. As a result, we squash and suppress our anger until it mutates into apathy, listlessness, and depression. When we deny a basic human emotion such as anger, our inner tapestry changes. We begin to shut down. We begin to shrivel and wither away.

What we don't realize when we suppress our anger is that we bury our vital right to claim our boundaries and own our space. When we are afraid of anger, in essence we declare that we are afraid of our power. In this small but profound manner, we allow our space and body to be violated.

Anger is a powerful messenger, alerting us to when something is wrong and needs to be corrected. The key to this is to respond, not react. Anger has a place in our lives, but we need to understand how to harness its power wisely. We need to consider how to *use* our head instead of *losing* our head.

Anger is a natural response in this unnatural world we live in. With so many outrageous indignities being conducted against humanity, how can we not experience anger? The key is not to resist the anger but, instead, to channel it into constructive action. Anger fuels us to take action. When we allow this fueling to be unobstructed, it can create massive change in our lives.

We need to create a new relationship to our anger. By owning and claiming its power, women begin to move away from our soft, feminine energy to occupy a stronger, more dominant masculine energy. We have been conditioned to think that being masculine is bad. But this is not true at all. Masculine energy, especially for "nice" girls, is the element they need to develop in order to stand tall and strong in their feeling center.

A healthy masculinity understands the power of *no* and uses it whenever necessary. Women who are able to integrate their feminine with their masculine are able to stand powerfully in their "no" energy without feeling compromised. They are able to use this power to check the men in their lives and stop them from entering a toxic masculinity. Such a woman never allows herself to be manipulated, exploited, dominated, controlled, or tyrannized. Men who are not able to handle her power will not be the enlightened ones she needs to surround herself with. The more she realizes this, the more the toxic relationships in her life will fade away.

Both our feminine and our masculine sides are pivotal aspects of the self that need to blossom. Traditionally, we have been scorned when we are more masculine and labeled as a "bitch," while men have been labeled as "sissies" for being more feminine. Thanks to the #metoo movement, a new way of regarding one another is currently coming to the fore. We are now occupying our masculine side with greater freedom, as men also claim their feminine side.

A healthy masculinity has nothing to do with domination over another but involves assertively aligning with one's own right to thrive. As we integrate our masculine, we begin to value who we are without being a watered-down version of ourselves. We boldly and unapologetically embrace our dreams and daringly pursue our destiny.

Embracing our masculine energy doesn't mean we forsake our gentleness, our empathy, our sensitivity, or our giving. These are what make us uniquely women. We want to keep our essence, our heart, and our compassion. We want to continue to feel, cry, and share. Holding on to our love for community and interdependence is key.

Collectively Creating a New World

When we awaken, we give our men a chance to awaken as well. When we allow our men to get away with abusive, violent, and predatory behavior, we fail them and our children. When we refuse to allow men to continue their tyrannical ways, they realize they cannot get away with toxic behavior anymore. As their mothers, sisters, and daughters, we have the power to stop toxic masculinity in its tracks.

The traits of toxic masculinity are not just possessed by men. Many women can show up with these too, and this must be acknowledged. Many in lesbian relationships have also experienced this from their partner even though she is a female. There are many reasons for developing toxic masculinity, ranging from people's innate proclivities to their childhood conditioning and cultural indoctrination. No matter where or how it shows up, it must be recognized and resisted, just like toxic femininity should.

The way forward is through the rising of the collective awakened female. Once we band together, we will stop our unconscious men from being their own worst enemies. We will collectively step up and put a dam on the toxicity that exists. By being secure in ourselves, instead of hesitant, compromising, and equivocating, we teach our unconscious men how to respect our vast intelligence and potential for leadership. They may resist, but at the end of the road, the upheaval will be worthwhile.

The first thing that needs to happen is we need to check the unbridled unconsciousness and violence that men, particularly white men, exhibit as a whole. While men should hold their brothers accountable for their actions, this is equally the responsibility of those of us who have been oppressed. When the oppressed become strong, the hierarchy weakens. Dominance at the cost of another's subjugation is never true power but a vestige of hidden cowardice.

On a deeply intuitive level, the men have to know they have botched things up. They can see that our children are anxious and that the separation created by institutions that divide us is growing. If only women stopped competing with one another and, instead, rose together as a collective, we could turn the world right side up. The key lies in our collective rising. When we stand up for one another against the patriarchy, we will be able to put our men in their rightful place—by our side, not in front of us.

The power to unite the globe belongs to women who, by nature, are intuitive connectors. The feminine principle intuitively knows how to nurture and blossom. It allows the mother that exists in most women to expand, release, and surrender. In this way, we profoundly and perfectly mirror Mother Earth—life-giving, regenerative, and restorative.

By possessing a maternal heart, the woman innately reveres life and intuitively protects it. She might not have the physical strength of a man, but she surpasses his limitations by her expansive heart and mind, exuding a wisdom and compassion that beats with the same emotional rhythm as the earth. When she balances this amazing loving heart with a powerful masculinity, she not only creates life, she also destroys anything that prevents life from flourishing. Her masculinity allows her to expand her nurturing to include protective boundaries. She loves, but is not afraid to thwart, those who create toxic hatred.

When we rise up in our individual power and join together with all our risen sisters, women will design a new tomorrow, one where there is no hierarchy at all but, instead, a circle of sisters and brothers who each know their place along the continuum of life. Each will be aware of their unique power and honor the contribution the other plays in the global whole.

We have one earth and we are one species. We are ultimately one throbbing, interconnected, interdependent being. What affects one affects all. The separations based on religion, color, education, income, status, and beauty are illusions. The awakened know this. Now it is their turn to speak and be heard.

Part Five

AWAKENING

from the

MATRIX

19

Embracing Fearless Boundaries

She finally cleared her eyes of its cobwebbed veils
And crushed the generational debris obscuring her path
And stepped out of the shadows of her parents' fears
And entered the bright dawn of her tomorrow
Trepidatious at first. But then boldly, embracingly.

We are all addicts in our own ways. We are addicts to our attachments, be it to our roles, relationships, emotional patterns, possessions, or beliefs. Like alcoholics with their addictions, we too are completely enslaved to these attachments. Ask a religious person to let go of their attachment and see what resistance you get. Similarly, ask any person in a conflict to give up their point of view and you will see the degree of attachment they hold. We have been enslaved by our attachments for so long that we don't even realize their hold on us.

The first step in shedding our facades is to realize we have been in survivor mode most of our life. As long as our attachments have a hold on us, we are bound to them. Their ensnarement over us is so deep that we don't fully appreciate their power over us. We react against them constantly and don't even know we are doing so. Robotic and zombielike, we repeat the same patterns over and over.

How do we break free and occupy a new way of being? How do women, especially, enter a new emotional territory and shift our selfhood from one of servility to power? What does it mean to be in a female body? To be connected and engaged to our leadership, power, and governance? We have allowed ourselves to ignore our inner truth for so long that to follow it feels strange and risky, yet this is precisely what we need to do if we are to truly embrace our power.

To step out of survivor mode into awakened mode takes courage. It requires that we dare to make the shift from being externally focused to being internally driven. This means we need to awaken to our inner knowing. This takes practice.

Each time we confront an external reality, instead of being drawn toward it in our typical way, we do something radical—we pause and turn inward. Instead of blindly reacting according to conditioned patterns we ask: Why am I reacting this way? What do I truly feel in this moment and how can I express this inner truth? Through this inner awakening, we begin to cultivate our authentic voice. When it rings clearer and clearer, we take charge of our reality. We finally step into a new kind of power—a power that realizes that no matter what is going on in the external world, there are infinite ways to respond. These choices liberate us and free us to create new pathways and new destinies.

The single biggest practical step I took that changed my day-to-day interactions was to learn to pause and listen to my inner self. I made it my practice. As I began to awaken and notice just how much I was driven by external forces, I knew I couldn't trust my patterns anymore. I needed to disrupt them. The only way to disrupt them was to create a new pattern in their place. So I made it a practice to meditate daily.

Through meditation, I learned to turn my awareness inward. I learned to pause before I talked, checking in with how I felt. This became second nature—so much so that now if I am out of alignment with my inner self, I immediately feel alarm bells ringing. I feel myself enter into a panic state that tells me something is wrong. I realize I have fallen into an old pattern by playing a role that isn't in alignment with my true self. Each time I enter lack, scarcity, and fear, I feel my entire body tense up. I now know that these are the signs of old patterns at play. Where before I would have succumbed to the desire to react to these patterns, I can now pause and say to myself, "Ah, here is the pattern again," and watch it with my inner eye. Not being ruled by our old emotional patterns is singlehandedly the greatest liberation we can give ourselves.

Susie, a client of mine, comes to mind here. She can still remember the very first time she didn't react in her typical way during a conflict. She had been coming to me for therapy for over a year and it was the first time she shifted her patterns. It happened during a conflict with her girlfriend of many years. During a misunderstanding, things blew up and her friend hurled accusations at Susie. Ordinarily, Susie would have reacted back in an equally wild way. Yet for the first time Susie made another choice and entered quietude. She didn't say a word back. "I just finally got it, Dr. Shefali! I finally understood what you have been telling me about my self-worth! It doesn't depend on anyone but me!" Susie was elated by her first taste of inner authorship. It was a moment of epiphany indeed.

This was Susie's breakthrough—her first glimpse of freedom. She was able to unshackle herself from the other's validation and enter her own. Susie rapidly began making changes in other areas of her life. She had finally stepped into her own skin. This is the power we each have to disrupt old patterns and create new paths for ourselves.

I am aware that all this can feel daunting. On some levels, it cannot be helped because learning any new skill takes practice and awareness. It is a lifelong endeavor for sure. By getting to this page, you are already taking the small steps you need toward your burgeoning self. The next chapters will continue to illuminate the path forward.

As we start to check in with ourselves more instead of blindly reacting to the external world, we begin to tap into silence more. The silence we have known in the past came from subjugation and shame. Now, a new form of silence dawns in our lives—the silence that comes with awakening. This new silence speaks to grounding ourselves in our inner power. It is a silence born out of wise discernment, not out of fear of losing the other's love. These two kinds of silence mark the difference between our awakening and our somnolence.

When we pause and listen to our inner voice, we curate a new earth for ourselves, one where the outside begins to match the inside. Instead of letting the outside rule us, we now place our inner self front and center. She is the one we first seek counsel with and abide by. We listen to her as if she were the most important being on this earth, because she is. Because we deem our inner self valid and worthy, we only lean into those situations that resonate with our essence. All that doesn't resonate slowly fades away. We no longer tolerate environments that squelch our inner self. In this way, our external tapestry begins to change.

Holding ourselves worthy of validation and honor changes the entire foundation of our lives. Taking first place in our own lives is not a position we occupy with hubris but with humility, as we finally realize that it's only a self that loves herself first that can truly embody a loving embrace of all.

The Wisdom of Discernment

A large part of self-honor has to do with discernment. If there was one lesson I missed in life, it was to have discernment when it came to people and situations. All I learned was to be nice, kind, and loving. No one taught me to discern. If only someone had shown me that as much as a loving heart is precious, it's going to be trampled if it isn't tempered with discernment.

The manifestation of discernment is the setting of boundaries. But the process of discernment starts way before any boundary is ever created. It begins with our understanding of the concept of the "consciousness quotient." Discernment is the capacity to understand our own and another's consciousness quotient.

One of the fundamental pieces of awareness I was lacking while growing up was the awareness of how different every single person's level of consciousness is. I presumed that just because we were all sentient and relatively intelligent, we were of a similar consciousness. Oh, how wrong I was! It took me at least my entire thirties to realize it. It isn't true that everyone's heart is wide open, nor is it true that everyone is loving and compassionate. The key determinant is the person's consciousness quotient.

What this measures, in a nutshell, is how much self-awareness a person possesses. Self-awareness is the key factor in a person's awakening. If the person isn't self-aware, they cannot really be expected to be in an intimate relationship with another. This self-awareness doesn't emerge in a void. It's something we cultivate on a daily basis. It's a reflection of how much inner work we have done.

I realized over time that the qualities of empathy, compassion, activism, and interconnectivity are not universal qualities in people. They are qualities that are unique to those with a certain level of consciousness. It takes intelligence, willingness, and a high degree of emotional integration to exhibit these qualities. If the person doesn't want to pursue them, they are not going to have a high consciousness quotient.

Discernment is the capacity to understand our own and another's consciousness quotient. There isn't an objective metric for this, but it basically probes into the other's level of self-awareness. Once we understand this, we no longer expect the other to behave in a particular way just because it's something we desire. We now understand that they may simply not be able to do so. If their consciousness quotient is low, how can we expect them to have the awareness we seek?

While most of us have grown up chronologically, our emotional and consciousness quotients are pretty low. Most of us appear as if we are adults, but we are actually walking, talking toddlers having one tantrum after another. Realizing this about ourselves and our loved ones, while disheartening on one level, can also be freeing.

When we realize we have been expecting the other to behave as an adult when they are actually toddlers on the inside removes some degree of personalization and hurt we feel. Seeing the toddler parts within ourselves can allow us to own up to them and have compassion for ourselves and others. In this way, much unnecessary suffering can be mitigated.

I am reminded of a piece of Buddhist lore. A monk was taking a walk with an apprentice and was approached by a beggar who asked for money. The monk immediately gave him money. The apprentice praised him for his compassion and generosity. The next day, another beggar approached the monk for money. The monk told him to stop being lazy and find a job. The apprentice was puzzled and inquired why he treated the second beggar differently. The monk explained that he intuited that the first one was really in need, whereas the second one was asking out of laziness. It's this kind of discernment to which I refer.

Because not everyone is at the same point in their consciousness, acting toward everyone in the same way isn't wise. Each person requires a different response from us, just like parents respond differently to each of their children. Each child has a different temperament, requiring a different parental response. A one-size-fits-all approach is never wise. So it is with relationships.

Discernment is different from judgment. Judgment is typically a mental belief that another is lesser-than and ought to be different from who they are. Judgment is the scourge of humanity, leading to war, violence, and death. It's the basis of white supremacy and all sorts of evils that are caused when humans believe only their ways are the right ways. Based on separation and fear, a judgment mode seeks to divide and conquer.

Discernment doesn't look to dominate the other. It simply seeks a deeper understanding of the other's emotional and spiritual character. It realizes that each person is on their own journey. Recognizing and honoring this journey within each individual, discernment doesn't seek to change the other. It asks us to make a choice whether to continue our interaction. If we choose to move away, we do so with release and joy, not with spite or resentment.

With discernment, we realize our power in cocreating life and don't passively allow anyone to enter our life and influence us. We ferociously protect our inner territory with the zeal of a lioness protecting her cubs. We move away from being a passive recipient toward an active engager. We judiciously cull, vet, pluck, extract, glean, and select whom we spend our energy on. This is being realistic, not judgmental. People and projects have to pass muster and make the high grade we set for friendships. Our self-honor and self-worth keep us from granting anyone who doesn't share a similar consciousness from gaining access to our inner terrain. Gone are the days of placid acquiescence and compliance. Our experiences now create a conscious match with how we wish to feel.

This is what it means to become a conscious architect of our life. We shift from being hapless bystanders in our life to being architects who meticulously select the right bricks and mortar with which to create the foundation of our existence. This doesn't mean we won't still make mistakes. All it means is that we will be aware that these mistakes were done under the best consciousness we had available to us at that time. There are no regrets, only opportunities for growth.

To become our own strongest advocate isn't something that comes easily to women. We have long been bulldozed into believing we are not good enough, strong enough, or worthy enough. We have been trained to need others to advocate for us. We have been far too comfortable being a passenger in our own life.

When I began to honor myself more than I honored others, my entire life shifted. I know it sounds extremely self-absorbed and narrowly focused when I speak in these terms, but actually it's the opposite. The care I had been meting out to others in my life before I awoke came from a place of fear, hesitation, and avoidance. It wasn't based in genuine abundance and generosity. It originated from an inner state of dependency, need, and lack. I didn't realize that I was playing the *role* of giver as opposed to genuinely giving of myself.

As I began to wake up to the many roles I played and the masks I wore, I realized that my giving was coming out of an inner void. It was coming out of my ego and was my strategy to obtain validity and the approval of others. When I began to break this pattern and only give to others out of a place of joy instead of obligation or fear, everything began to change. Yes, I lost a lot of relationships. At first this was scary, but soon I realized these were relationships based on my false self's fear, as opposed to the power of my true self.

Post-awakening, I spent much time shedding my false masks and with them my false relationships. It was so hard for me to create boundaries and respect my own voice. Through my daily inner alignment, I was slowly able to move away from relationships that were false. I began to smell them a mile away and could avoid their ever taking root in my psyche. My desire to never compromise myself overrode my desire for friendship. A relationship either aligned with my truth or I chose to be alone.

When we reach this place of nonnegotiability, when we decide we will never give up our truth for anything, we align our outer world with our inner world. It's almost as if we give off a certain scent that others pick up. Those who cannot handle our truths naturally stay away. Only those who are on a similar path show up. Just making the decision to stand in our worth does the work for us.

Once we set the intention to honor our worth and our inner voice, we hold front-and-center the question, Does this match how I wish to feel? We envision a clear image of who we wish to be and how we wish to feel. We move away from situations that don't match this intention and move joyfully toward those that do.

Coming from a place of inner abundance and synchronicity, there is no longer an urgency or scarcity that causes us to glom on to the first opportunity that comes our way. We wait, pause, and allow the situation to percolate. We see how people and situations taste, touch, and sound. We wait for them to show their colors before we commit our heart and mind. In this way, we create a space for full alignment to take place before we declare a union with another.

The Art of Sacred Boundaries

Setting boundaries in our intimate relationships, saying no to those who might depend on us, and walking away from toxic dynamics are some things I always avoided. Now I realize that I was lying to myself. I realize I can never really be in an authentic relationship until I first come from a place of self-worth, self-honor, and self-advocacy. There is no way to save anyone else if we ourselves are drowning.

Creating boundaries means to say no, plain and simple. It is our way of saying, "This doesn't feel right to me and I need to stop participating in it." We either say no through our words or our actions. The no isn't to the other person, per se. It's to ourselves. We say no to the roles we have robotically and unconsciously played in the past. It's not about asking the other person to change. It just demands that we stop our participation in the dynamic.

Many of us have been confused with what the word *no* means. We think that to say no means we need to explain or justify ourselves or engage in conflict. Or we think it means we need to help the other make the changes we think they need to make. For these reasons, saying no feels onerous. But actually, it just means we've decided we are done. Done with what? Our engagement. This is what ends when we start saying no. It has nothing to do with the other. All it means is that we are shutting off our lights and turning down our energy. We disengage. Whatever it was that we were doing to keep the dynamic going, we stop. In essence, we say "no" to the little girl within us that desires approval, validation, and praise. We tell her this: "You do not need these crumbs of worth from the other person anymore. You are already whole and complete within. Do not be afraid to step into this inner power."

For the first part of our awakening journey, we may find that we need to say no all the time. The more we have been asleep in our relationships, allowing ourselves to be surrounded by dysfunction, the more we need to weed this out of our life. The more we become conscious, the more we will need to say "no."

The more junk food we ate before, the more we will need to say "no" to our senses till they detox from their usual compulsions. The more "junk" relationships we had, the more we will need to do the same here, too. At first, it will feel like we are constantly saying "no" to ourselves, and this will feel restrictive. But this is not so. We are loving ourselves for the first time in our life. The more we construct a dam to the toxic elements of our life, the more we open the waterways for a joyful flood of health and abundance.

A large part of sacred boundaries involves clarifying our limits. What are our limits around words spoken to us? What words are acceptable and what words are not? What about the tone of speech? What about the behavior? Our mothers may never have taught us to create limits around how people act toward us and this may have led us to believe they aren't necessary. Only when women have a clear vision of how we need to be treated will we teach others the same. If we don't know what these limits are, how will others figure it out?

Setting boundaries is not the act of a selfish person but the act of a *selfless* person. When we make our boundaries clear to others, we aren't only taking care of ourselves but also them. Everyone needs a guidebook to who we are and how we would like to be treated. Clear boundaries give us this guidebook. "I don't ever like to be spoken to like this, so please be aware" is not a nasty thing to say but a kind thing.

Part of laying out sacred boundaries and creating matched alignments within our relationships means to dare to create these with our family of origin. This is the ultimate frontier in the realm of sacred boundary making. Although someone may be family, they may not be "our people." Making the distinction between those we have no conscious choice but to relate to and those we can now consciously include in our lives marks the arrival of the awakened woman. Breaking free from the tentacles of family, we design a new life where each person raises us toward our highest potential.

When we don't create these boundaries against the toxic elements in our life, we communicate consent toward them. Realizing that our silence is indirect complicity is a crucial realization as we become awakened. Simply feeling bad is not enough. We need to communicate this to the external world by either emotionally or physically leaving a situation. This requires us to transfer our feelings into action. Here is where we move from the feminine into the masculine. When we do, we make our viewpoint known and our voice heard. Sure, this might cause an unwarranted ripple effect, which is precisely what we dread, but we must ask the inevitable question: What do I fear?

Most women don't create boundaries because we imagine some terrible future consequence, such as being rejected, deserted, invalidated, financially crippled, or shamed in some way. We imagine the worst, and this projection keeps us silenced and withdrawn. What we don't realize is that what we fear has already occurred in some way, shape, or form.

When I feared actually going through a divorce, I imagined being alone and bereft. It was only when I hunkered into my own being that I came to see that I was already alone and bereft in many ways. I was already lacking the intimacy I was afraid of being without in the future. My fear about the future had already manifested in the present moment. What could be worse than what had already occurred?

So it is in all of our lives. We imagine a terrible future without realizing that this fear of the future comes from events already occurring or that have occurred in the past. In fact, it's from our past that we glean evidence for the future. If the past hadn't occurred the way it did, we wouldn't be imagining the future. The most beautiful thing about future planning is that there are literally infinite possibilities. No matter how we plan it, we can never fully plan it exactly the way it will happen.

I always ask my clients, "Is your *now* palatable? If it is not, don't worry about the future. First, accept that the present is unbearable." We must work to create health and well-being in the *now*. It makes no sense to worry about what tomorrow will bring when today is already toxic. It's like wanting to wait a few days to put out the fire even though it's going to burn the house down right here, right now.

Awakened women have a lot to express—not because we desire to be noisy for the sake of attention, but because we are living, breathing citizens of this world who are affected by events around us. We are curious, engaged, and caring. We will not be a pushover anymore nor will we be silenced. We know our voice must be heard and are not going to be shy in expressing it.

Nothing matters more than our inner state. As we fine-tune our inner synchrony, we become more seasoned at discerning toxic elements in the world around us. Soon our entire life shifts into a near-perfect manifestation of this inner harmony. We begin to live life from the inside out. We taste what it means to be empowered and free.

~

20

Embracing Sovereignty

For years she lived behind cowardly shadows
Afraid to ruffle their feathers and anger them
Tiptoeing, she learned to walk with stealth and quiet
Until one day something changed and she no longer feared them
It was only here that the maid morphed into the Queen.

If there is one word most women hate, it's being called a "bitch." I certainly did. I ranted and raved each time I was called that. I felt the need to justify myself, imploding and exploding. It was only when I realized the reason I was being called a *bitch* had nothing to do with me and had everything to do with whether I was capitulating to another that I stopped resisting the word. I began to see how we have been afraid of this word, seeing it as a personal derogation when, in fact, it's a sign of our power.

I'm not advocating that this become common parlance, just that we understand what this word really implies. My point is, when we are called a *bitch*, it's not about us at all. It's all to do with how *un*submissive and powerful we actually are. This word is an acknowledgment of our sovereign autonomy.

The US feminist magazine *BITCH* explains it like this on its website: "When it's being used as an insult, bitch is an epithet hurled at women who speak their minds, who have opinions and do not shy away from expressing them and who do not sit by and smile uncomfortably if they are bothered or offended. If being an outspoken woman means being a *bitch*, we will take that as a compliment, thanks."

The more we honor our voices and claim our power, the more we are going to be called a *bitch*. Culture doesn't like empowered women who speak up for themselves. Calling us *bitches*, *sluts*, or *whores* is one of the ways culture controls its powerful women. When we understand this, we stop taking these words personally. We understand that pissing people off comes with the territory. When people are pissed off, they seek to silence the other using shaming terms. After all, how dare we change the rules of the game! Everyone was used to our meekness and silence. And now? How dare we think we can start changing things?

The moment we start laying out our boundaries and acting in accord with our inner voice, we are going to hear all sorts of backlash. *Where did that lovely girl go?* they will say. *Why are you being such a bitch?* These words may feel like thorns in our sides. All our lives, we worked so hard to be lovely and not be "the bitch," so they know exactly what our Achilles' heel is.

If we are still attached to our image as the "good" one, we feel a huge inner uprising when we experience invalidation from others. We flounder, flail, and storm within. We don't know which way to turn. We begin to second-guess ourselves and wonder, "Maybe I should have just said yes? Maybe then they would still like me the same way." It's here that another fork in the road presents itself: do we want to be authentic or do we want to be loved?

Enter the Queen

When we are attached to receiving a stream of validation and love from the other, we literally desert our truth in order to be in their favor. Until this addiction of wanting the other to endorse us is healed, we will never own our sovereign truth. A large part of this healing involves tolerating others' disapproval, disdain, and contempt for us. How do we get to the place of releasing people who don't honor or celebrate us? It sounds so ruthless, so cold. What are the mental shifts we need to make in order to arrive at this place?

It begins by leaving behind our damsel Princess energy and entering our empowered Queen energy. We need to move from passive to active, dependent to independent, weak to empowered. This can only happen when we begin to love ourselves.

Let me explain what "loving ourselves" means to me. It means that the love we get from ourselves is *more valuable* than the love we receive from another. This is key. The feeling we get when we honor ourselves needs to be more of a bejeweled treasure than the feeling we get when another honors us. When we arrive at the place where our own self-approval and self-validation matter more than that of others, we turn to ourselves for wise counsel, like we would have previously turned to a wise leader in the past. Instead of calling a friend on the phone, we call on our inner self. When we are sad, we accompany ourselves on a journey inward to discover the reason. When we are happy, we celebrate ourselves and experience inner pride without the need for outer approval.

Getting used to being alone is a large part of the awakening process. Preferring to be on one's own rather than being with those of a differing consciousness emerges naturally. Where before our own company may have terrified us, now we welcome it. This displacement of others as our top priority allows us to stop caring what they think. It isn't as if we don't invite feedback from them; it's just that we don't blindly prostrate ourselves before it. We pause, look within, and discern whether the opinion of others overrides what we think. When we do, we have arrived in our Queen energy.

When I speak of the Queen, I don't mean to evoke the tyrant who cuts off people's heads. I speak of The Awakened Queen, one who works from her heart as well as her mind, her receiving as well as her giving. She is fully settled into her worth and desires nothing more than to empower others to know theirs as well.

The Queen is never cut off from her heart. In fact, she is fully grounded in it. She sees how others operate from lack and has compassion for them. Instead of being threatened by others' anxieties or influenced by them, she stands strong in her own wisdom. She builds her queendom of carefully selected women who, like her, are past living in separation or fear.

The Queen is the archetype of a woman who is no longer apologetic about her inner right to take up space and hold court. She is no longer ambivalent about her capacity to contribute and make a difference. She is no longer afraid to shine. She is fully and irrevocably aware of her worth and no longer cowers in the shadows afraid to display herself as boldly as she desires.

The Queen no longer sees herself as lesser-than—ever. She fully sees herself as an equal at the table, be it a table of peasants or presidents. Because she has seen through the illusion of labels and identification, she is no longer intimidated. She doesn't need to be the most credentialed, the most glamorous, or the wealthiest to take her place at the table. She sits at the table because she fully and wholly recognizes that she is worthy just as she is.

No longer beguiled by fancy suits and diamond bracelets, she cuts through the blind illusions of cultural indoctrinations. She is here to show up for herself—curious, openhearted, and present. If another doesn't value this, she moves on without a grudge or even a care. She knows the ocean is vast and there will be many who will match her. She no longer seeks approval or validation, for to do so would be to stoop below her worth.

The Queen values her own voice so much that she places herself in a position of great honor. No one comes before her. She doesn't fall under the spell of another's power before her own. She has broken that spell. She now fully realizes that she has her own power to turn to, her own inner compass to guide her, and her own resources to count on. The damsel in distress has woken up and is no longer dependent on her prince. The Prince fantasy is charred, dead, and buried.

When I began to enter my Queen energy, I immediately experienced a backlash from my loved ones. The most common retort was, "Who does she think she is?" I am sure many women have heard this. What this question means is: How dare you place yourself before me? And, How dare you think so highly of yourself that you don't care more about my needs?

When women hear this question, we subconsciously feel admonished, as if we have been called to the principal's office for a scolding. We have stepped out of line and are going to pay for it. The more we have set up past dynamics of servitude to others' needs before our own, the more we are going to fear this backlash. We are afraid to dare, you see. We associate daring with badness. "Only bad girls dare." These doubts are intended to stop us from daring, to keep us in our place, to keep us silenced. When I realized that this was a bully tactic, I stopped flinching when I heard these words. I trained myself to look straight at the person meting them out and hold their gaze without fear.

Only when I was able to own and accept *Hell, yeah, I place myself first and you better believe I think highly of myself* was I able to leave my helpless inner damsel behind. When we women begin to think of ourselves as daring and majestic, we give others no choice but to think of us in the same light. Why should others think of us as amazing or worthy if we are constantly shying away from this light? We need to stop cowering in fear, reeling in shame, and waiting in passivity. We need to wake up and believe we are competent, capable, and savvy as hell. Head held high, shoulders broad, we begin to manifest the power we have always had within us.

I remember a moment when I stepped into my own Queen energy. It happened during my conference, Evolve, where one of the participants ranted at me about how this conference was a waste of her money. As she attacked me, one part of me wanted to capitulate and apologize. I wanted to refund her money and assuage her pain. Thankfully, there was another part—my Queen part. This part was completely fine with her displeasure and invalidation. This part understood it was not about me. Why? Because I believed in myself and didn't need her to validate who I was. Also, this part saw through her words to another part of her—her pain. I invited her onstage to work through her reactions. As expected, once all her feelings came out, it was clear I was just a target for her inner conflicts, and that all her "attacks" were really about her own inner state of dishevelment.

When we remember our own true worth by channeling our inner Queen, we are able to separate who we are from another's beliefs about us. This "stepping into worth" is a key ingredient in our growth. It is what the Queen does with ease.

The No-Excuse Zone

If there is one question I have now sworn to obliterate from my quiver, it's, Why are you being so mean to me? I have sworn never to ask the question "why" if it has to do with ill-treatment toward me. For decades I used to wonder about the "why" of a person's behavior as if there was some justification that would make a person's behavior toward me acceptable. It was as if the bad behavior was tolerable if it had a justifiable cause. What this really meant was that the other's state of mind and heart was more important than the hurt and pain they caused me.

It was only after I woke up that I realized there was no "why" that was good enough at the end of the day, except, "I am unconscious and I need to work on myself." All other reasons were justifications for their ill-treatment of me and a distraction from the fact that I needed to create a no-excuse zone against such treatment.

The bottom line is that there is no acceptable reason for ill-treatment from myself or others. This fact took a while to sink in. Each time my persona of empath popped up, trying to be a savior or rescuer, I gently shoved her back down. I didn't allow her to second-guess me. I valued her beautiful heart, but I knew that until I created new conditions for her to blossom, she would need to stay quiet. It was not the time for my empathic side to shine. It was time for my Queen to rise.

So afraid are we to own our feelings that women constantly seek permission from the outside world. It's almost as if we need a reason before we follow our own intuition. It's as if our feelings are never enough. We need to know the other's reason first. If the other's reason is big enough or strong enough, then we are willing to squash ours down.

Right here, we once again see our fundamental problem as caring and nurturing women. We care for the wounds and feelings of others much more than we do our own. Don't get me wrong—there is nothing wrong in expressing our love for others. It's our most wonderful quality. But it can become toxic when we place that quality over self-love and self-care.

When I realized I did this not so much because I cared for the other but because I was scared to care for myself, I knew something was wrong. It was wrong to believe I wasn't as important as anyone else. It was wrong to believe my feelings weren't important just as they are. It was time to change these beliefs, and I did so by stepping into my Queen.

I began to create a no-excuse zone around me. I stopped making excuses for other people or myself. I stopped saying "because" and simply started saying "It is what it is." No "because," no reason, no excuse. If the behavior toward me was unacceptable, I stopped searching for the deeper meaning. I allowed myself the privilege of simply saying, "I will not be treated in this way. End of story."

So guided is the Queen by her inner truth that following its beacon is her only concern. The guiding question is simple: Does it feel good to me? If it does, take another step forward. If it doesn't, let it go. Feeling deserving of all good things is difficult for us self-sacrificing women, but it is what we need to step into if we are to fully own our inner sovereignty. The Queen understands that she is:

Deserving of space to be big and loud
Deserving of respect and celebration
Deserving of patience and loyalty
Deserving of attention and validation
Deserving of indulgent care
Deserving of truth and honesty

Deserving of wealth and material comforts if she has worked for
  them
Deserving of luxury and enjoyment if it comes her way
Deserving of receiving lavish praise and adoration
Deserving of being in the spotlight if it shines on her
Deserving of being loved and honored
Deserving of self-care and relaxation

The Queen doesn't doubt that she is self-deserving. She wears her crown and sits on her throne with a regal inner knowing. A true Queen feels so secure in her own inner power that she is comfortable allowing others to rise to their Queen nature as well. This is where the ultimate power of the Queen is found. She creates the space for others to flourish. So fulfilled is she from her own journey toward wholeness, she effortlessly creates the space for others to feel secure to discover theirs. She never feels the need to compete or tread on anyone else's feet because hers are wearing golden shoes.

The Queen isn't waiting to be someone else before she can love herself. She realizes that she will always be a work in progress, but she is fully worthy of being honored and celebrated just as she is. Unlike the Princess, who keeps waiting for a brighter future, the Queen refuses to be in stall mode ever again. She realizes that life is lived in the present moment. No matter how messy or incomplete, it's who she needs to be at this point in time.

The Queen doesn't hide from her flaws but stakes her claim to them. She doesn't pretend to be all put together like a perfect gift, but bares her wounds for all to see. She is in touch with her shadow energy. Instead of letting her imperfections hide behind cobwebs, she owns them.

The Right Match

The Queen carefully selects her co-Queens and Kings. As she holds her time valuable, she just doesn't waste it on just anyone who desires her attention. She is willing to turn people away if they don't match with her consciousness.

What I am about to say is an extremely important lesson to teach our daughters. I wish I had known this before embarking on adulthood. When a woman fully claims her Queen energy, she stops chasing the attentions of the men or women around her. On the contrary, she waits for them to suit her and picks only the worthiest mates for herself. The Queen waits for the match to arrive. She doesn't go seeking it out of desperation or lack. She is secure in her knowledge that all things appear at the right time. There is no rush within her. She has lost her hustle, her thirst, her hunger. Whatever she needs lies right here, within her. There is no longing or craving to do or be anything other than what shows up in the moment.

As more of us step into our own inner royalty, we will pave the way for others to do so. It starts with one woman. As lonely as she may feel, it takes only one to start the revolution.

21

Embracing Accountability

I will no longer be the victim of my circumstances
No longer washed astray by the tide of my life
No longer broken by the winds of my storm
There is no one to blame, no one to wait for
It is time for me to take the helm and steer the ship.

Accountability is a pivotal aspect of our spiritual awakening. It means we are ready to be responsible for ourselves—fully. We end the blame-game and move away from a victim consciousness where we believe life is happening *to* us. Taking accountability for ourselves means we move into the awareness that life is happening *with* us.

When parents ask me how they can best apologize to their children, I often say, "Don't say you're sorry if you aren't going to be accountable." What I mean by this is that our children don't need to hear an empty sorry followed by a justification. All they care about is real change.

We are always "under contract." What do I mean by this? The emotional patterns we are bound by set up attachments within us that we then adhere to, as we would a contract. We enter contracts of martyrdom, victimhood, and anxiety. One of the major contracts we undertake unconsciously is the avoidance of responsibility. We are terrified of breaking this contract. To do so would mean ending all the childish tactics we employ. The question we need to ask ourselves is not whether we are ready to be joyful, but rather are we ready to break our "avoidance of responsibility" contract.

What would this look like in real life? To begin with, it would demand that we ask ourselves the following questions:

How did I contribute to my current situation?
What were my actions and behavior?
What emotional contract am I playing right now and why?
Why am I falling prey to old patterns?
What do I need to change to ensure that this pattern is disrupted?
How am I going to ensure that I create these changes?
What will I do in case of relapse?

Just as alcoholics need to take their addictions seriously, so too do we need to take our emotional addictions seriously. When we do a careful analysis of what leads us to fall prey to our unconscious emotional contracts, we ask: What are the causes I have created and the effects that came from this? What are my key triggers? What are the reactions in the body?

Observing the moment-by-moment, play-by-play of our causes and effects helps us see where the emotional fissures occurred. Just like a seismologist might do when recording an earthquake, we create a record of our inner turbulence. In this way, we begin to see exactly how the same patterns keep repeating themselves, and we can concertedly start breaking our dysfunctional contracts.

When we decide to take accountability, we declare to ourselves and others that no one is expected to take care of us anymore. This doesn't mean we don't appreciate being cared for. It means we no longer wait and hope for a knight in shining armor to come to our rescue. We fully embrace our own power to make the changes we need and start taking the steps to do so. In this way, the toddler not only begins to walk, she begins to fly.

The Allure of Unjust Justifications

"I ate the cookies because I was in such a bad mood all day!"

"I lost my temper because my kid was just not listening to me!"

"I understand why he hits me sometimes. I can really be a difficult person."

"I just wish he wasn't a workaholic. My life would be so different then."

Any of these sound familiar? We are master justifiers. Conditioned to avoid shame and punishment, we have learned to find justifications for our own and others' actions. Justifications are the main way we stay stuck in dysfunctional patterns, be it unhealthy relationships or jobs. Even though we may know we are unhappy, we continue to remain in these situations. The main reason is because we have justified the reason to remain.

Creating justifications is the opposite of accountability. Justifications passively generate excuses for why we or another did or didn't do something. Accountability actively creates actions to change the situation as soon as possible. One is replete with stagnant energy, the other with adaptive resilience.

Blame is a common way we create justifications. We point a finger at either ourselves or another and find reason to punish or judge. We stay in victim consciousness, either cowering in unworthiness if we blame ourselves, or cowering in disempowerment if we blame someone else for our current situation. Blame creates shame and fear of retribution.

One of the other ways we create justifications is through *cognitive dissonance reductions*. A term coined by psychologist Leon Festinger, it implies a psychological process where we try to reduce the discrepancy between two conflicting beliefs. If a woman is being ill-treated by her partner, she experiences a discomfort between two of her beliefs: her partner loves her, and ill-treatment is unacceptable. What is she to do now? She tries to reduce the discrepancy by changing one of her beliefs. Either she changes the belief that he loves her or she changes her definition of ill-treatment. In this way, she creates a new reality for herself by either leaving him or changing her views on the ill-treatment such that she no longer sees it as unacceptable.

Blame and cognitive dissonance reductions keep us from taking the giant leap we need if we are to "adult up" and take accountability for our life.

Justifications keep us stuck at the mental level of dashed hopes, unfulfilled wishes, incomplete ideas, and unmet fantasies. Accountability means we stop construing and constructing mental stories and start taking concrete action instead. We stop giving our power away and start creating positive steps toward change.

Moving into Empowered Action

Accountability is one of the final frontiers of becoming a true adult—not just chronologically but psychologically and emotionally. To "adult up" involves the absolute understanding that we are the creators of our mental states and inner realities. While we cannot always control our outer reality, we are in full control of our inner world.

This is one of my writings on accountability I have on my board in my office to remind me, and in turn my clients, where my problems and the solutions lie:

> *Everything I see comes from my own mind*
> *Everything I feel comes from my own mind*
> *Everything I know others to be comes from my own mind*
> *When I am broken, I interpret the other's brokenness as mine*
> *When I am whole, I interpret the other's brokenness as theirs.*

Reality is always neutral, neither good nor bad. This is hard to wrap our minds around. Many times we believe that reality is begging us to interpret it in a certain way, but this is just coming from our conditioning. The reason most of us cannot even explore alternate interpretations of reality is that our reactions are so knee-jerk, they don't feel as if they emerged from us. They feel as if they emerged from the reality itself.

The next step after awareness is action. What action steps do I need to take so that I am not in the same spiral again? How can I make sure I recognize my triggers in the moment and create a new way of being? This is where we show ourselves and those we have hurt that we are willing to shift in real time. We demonstrate that we are not speaking empty words.

Accountability is an act of great courage. It requires an inner time-out from our thoughts about reality. This kind of mental detachment doesn't come easily. It needs to be cultivated. The way I attempt to cultivate detachment is through meditation, during which I allow myself to step back from my thoughts into the place of observer. In this way, I create an inner space that now exists between my outer and inner world. This inner space is a third space. In this third space, I am no longer a reactor. I now have the potential to be a manifester.

Meditation is a powerful tool I employ to learn and practice detachment, and I strongly recommend that you begin to cultivate it in your life as well. The reason why I am a firm believer in it is because it helps us disrupt our incessant thinking and refocuses our minds on the present moment. Even if for five minutes at a time, I would recommend you use one of the many free meditation apps online and start your practice today.

Conscious Manifestation

We are always manifesting. Our manifestation is just not yet under our conscious and intentional control. The way to consciously enter our manifestation potential is to start to fully invest in observing and awakening to our inner reality.

As long as we believe that our outer reality has power over our inner reality, we will stay dependent on it, forever hoping that it stays positive so we can stay positive too. Only when we understand that our inner reality exists on a dimension quite separate from our outer reality do we finally grow up and take charge of our destiny.

To enter into our power as conscious manifesters doesn't mean we start wishing upon stars and dreaming up all sorts of fantasies. It has nothing to do with sticking pictures of Bentleys or private beaches on our bulletin boards. What it really means is that we become the conscious curators of what goes on our inner bulletin board. What thoughts are we going to stick up there? What interpretations? What belief systems and attachments? Instead of working from the outside in, we work from the inside out. We first take care of what is going on within and then look to how the outside world can or cannot support this.

It takes a great deal of emotional and spiritual work for us to realize that our inner reality can lead the way, influenced by the outer but not acting as its blind servant. We can hold on to our inner truth and simply not care as much about what the outer reality dictates. When we realize we hold dominion over our inner world, we taste what it means to be a conscious manifester. We understand what spiritual detachment is and begin to shed our enmeshment with our outer world.

As we design our inner bulletin boards, the first big piece of this work is releasing old news items. All old columns and expired tabloids need to be incinerated. This in itself is a process. For example, if we want to consciously manifest a healthier body, the first step is to throw out all the junk food from our cupboards.

We then go deeper and we begin to prioritize our inner worlds. Now we do another process of discernment. What matters most to us? And we create a ladder of priorities. Then, step-by-step, we articulate a trajectory for change.

Unless we go through this careful culling process, we are likely to get overwhelmed and not know where to begin. It's like going to a hoarder's house and not knowing where to start the removal process. So it is with our minds. We have been hoarding so much unconscious garbage in there that we need many days and lots of patience to go through the years of accumulated baggage.

Accountability in our adult relationships requires that we detach from the expectation that *any* of our personal needs will be met by the other *unless proven otherwise*. I realize this sounds cold and jaded, but it isn't. It is actually full of wisdom. No one can simply be expected to meet our needs unless two conditions are met—the first is that they are physically and emotionally able to, and they are willing and wanting to do so.

When the other is able to fulfill these two conditions, then something strange happens. Our needs begin to melt, opening up opportunities for connection and further evolution. But until these two conditions are present, we need to engage our inner adult and inner parent, giving *ourselves* what we seek from the outside world. In short, we take full charge of all the screaming children within us that are nothing more than memories of what happened to us in the past. One scab at a time, we address these memories. We need to recognize that when something in our external world brings back these memories, that's all they are—memories. We are adults now, not children. So the next time we believe someone has hurt us, we pause. Before we lash out in blame, we instead turn inward and ask ourselves: How are my old wounds causing me to interpret this situation in this way right now?

Taking accountability means taking ownership of our inner world and all its demons, wounds, and inadequacies. If you have trouble separating your adult self from past hurt, you may need the help of a therapist, coach, or good friend. This is absolutely essential at times. Asking for help is the action we need to take to begin the hard journey of healing ourselves. However, a word of caution. Beware that many in the helping professions are locked into their own past as if they themselves were still children. You don't need someone who will allow you to wallow in what happened—you need someone who will help you see what happened for what it is, your past.

Taking accountability doesn't mean wallowing. It just means waking up to how our past influences the present and absolving the present moment of blame. It literally means that we say to ourselves, "I am creating my own stress, my own anxieties, my own powerlessness. No one on the outside is doing this, just me." That's how radical this is.

We don't realize the power we can have over our own mind. If only we did, we would never need to withdraw from our heart in anger or pain. It's because we have given our power away that we react without any awareness of our part. We act as if we are tethered to the outer person or situation, like a puppet to its puppeteer. We need to realize there are no strings—none. They don't exist. Any that appear are figments of our imagination. There is no one out there that holds any power over us other than what we choose to give them. Once we fully embrace this, we truly step into our freedom and power. The question we always return to is, Am I ready?

22

Embracing Purpose

Just as the sun is ever flowing with its light
So is your purpose ever flowing within you
It isn't something to be found or searched for
It is right there, deep within you, longing for expression
It emerges when you are present to your truth.

It seems as if everyone is teaching a "find your purpose" course. We create vision boards with things we believe would give us purpose and strive to attain what's on them. Some of us believe our purpose is to be happy, while others believe that it's our purpose to be successful. Or perhaps we think it's to become a mother or a husband. Whatever it is, it's something outside of us—something we can get, hold on to, collect, and grow, like a collection of marbles. This is our first mistake when it comes to identifying our purpose.

Purpose is a state of being. As such, it's the fabric of our existence, the net that contains all things, relationships, and situations. It's the sinewy muscles of every experience and every breath we take. In essence, it's who we authentically are—a being of purpose.

There Is Nothing to Be Found

A common belief is that our purpose is something that needs to be found. This is a lie. Our purpose is always within us. What's missing is not purpose, per se, but our connection to it. This disconnection comes from our inner misalignment right here, right now. As long as we aren't aligned with the deepest, most authentic aspect of our being in the present moment, we will feel disconnected. As long as we are disconnected, we will be disengaged on some level. As long as we are disengaged, we will not tap into our purpose even though it's staring us in the face.

If we are living from our false self, purpose will never be found in the next job or the next relationship. We may find more wealth and status, or greater identification with the roles we play, but once these wear thin we will be back to square one. This is why those vision boards filled with fancy cars, vacations, and homes are a smokescreen—a misguided strategy that takes us further and further from the truth of who we are. Instead of chasing things, places, or people, we need to sit still and go deep within to ask: Is who I am in alignment with my most natural self? Is what I'm doing right now a match for how I truly feel?

Let's remove the superficialities from our vision boards and replace them with these pivotal questions:

Who am I today? Is this woman my truest self right now?
Who am I *not* today? Can I leave these qualities behind for good?
What do I want more of in my life so I can be authentic?
What do I *not* want in my life anymore so I can be authentic?
What can I do in this moment to arrive at a new inner state?

When we focus on these pivotal self-growth questions day in and day out, our intention and attention shift from finding something on the outside to fulfill us to searching deep within. As we go inward and shift away from people, places, and situations that cause us to become inauthentic and toward those that make us more authentic, we automatically enter a greater alignment with ourselves. Now, from this place of inner alignment, making an egg, cleaning our child's diaper, or singing a song all feel purposeful. The real ingredient of purpose turns out to be engagement and connection, which we cannot have without authenticity.

We can be doing the most amazing thing in the world, but if we are not engaged or connected with it, it eventually becomes meaningless. This is the reason for finding our *why*. If our why doesn't match our what, we will never feel purposeful. This is why inner work is the key pathway to purpose. Through this work, purpose is something we are and become.

In order to understand where purpose is found, it's imperative we understand the nature of purpose. What are its elements and how can we recognize it when it reveals itself within us?

The Magic of Presence

Purpose and life are inextricable. As long as we are alive, we have a purpose. At the most basic level, our purpose is to stay and feel alive. This can only be done when we are engaged with who we are moment-by-moment. When we lose connection with ourselves in the moment, we lose our capacity to feel alive and our sense of purpose disappears. The moment we are connected and present to ourselves in the here and now, purpose appears. Purpose, then, is one thing only—presence.

Contrary to common belief, purpose isn't relegated to the lucky or the privileged. It's something that each of us has within, and it calls for our recognition and commitment to this truth. Hence our purpose can only emerge when we are awake and present.

Purpose is presence and presence is authenticity and inner connection. Each of these feeds the other. They are overlapping circles connected at their core. We cannot separate them. Sadly, the self-help movement has failed to understand this interrelation and has parsed purpose and presence out as if they are separate from each other.

When we understand the interconnectedness of all things, we begin to birth a new relationship to purpose. We no longer ask, What is my purpose? but instead ask, What are the barriers to my true self? We now realize that as long as we stay in our false self, we will stay disembodied from our purpose. We understand that when we are connected to our truth, we are purposeful, no matter what we are doing. Our greatest purpose is to be true to ourselves.

We have been sold the idea that purpose is a *doing* state, involving achievement, success, wealth, motherhood, or career goals. These have little to do with true purpose. When we are fed the idea that these elements give us purpose, we once again chase the wrong rainbow and end up distracted and disillusioned. We believe there's something wrong with us. When we realize we have been sold yet another bag of goods, we realize that the true prize can never be found in the doing, only in the being. It is here that we understand the jewel of life: true purpose is the child of the authentic self. Coming home to ourselves is the ultimate goal of life.

Purpose and presence are interchangeable and can never be torn apart. Each is inextricably married to the other. And what is the offspring they birth? *Meaning.*

Once we seek to manifest our true self at every juncture through presence and purpose, every moment begins to be infused with a quality that's deep and profound. Now everything has meaning. Nothing is an isolated, random event. Everything has a deeper meaning to us because we are tuned into everything, as a student would be to their teacher. We see every moment as a mirror to a deeper lesson that we need to learn. As such, meaning abounds everywhere. We keep asking ourselves: What is this moment here going to teach me? We know there is always a purpose and are on the lookout in terms of uncovering meaning. In this way, our lives are never meaningless, random, or wasted. Every moment is alive and replete with a lesson and the potential for growth.

Soon the implicit purpose we see everywhere begins to take root as a manifested purpose—a purpose we can now activate as a goal and put into action. We cannot help but radiate our inner connection in an outward and palpable manifestation. As we keep looking inward and deeper, we move closer to our true self and begin to drop the people, behavior, and situations that do not match this true self, moving toward those that do.

Now we begin doing things that light us up and give us joy. No longer do we waste time in endeavors that create dissonance. Over time, we find ourselves more and more rooted in activities and behavior that induce direct passion and joy. Before we know it, we are engaged in our manifested purpose.

Purpose is uncovered from the inside out, not the other way around.

A New Embrace of Purpose

Upon awakening, I began to realize that every moment is infused with purpose. Until then, I just hadn't realized this. So attached was I to how things needed to look on the outside that I was looking in all the wrong places. I thought purpose needed to look a certain way.

Now I see that purpose is not in *how things look*, but in *how I look at things*.

Once I realized how rife with purpose every moment is, I began to "make love" to all of my life experiences—my writing, my relationships, my speaking, my cooking, my exercising, and my parenting. In each of these moments, I paid homage to my purpose. As I embraced my present moment, I embraced my connection to it and, through this, my purpose. The present moment became the gift, not the adornments that wrapped it.

When I am in a state of lack, the present moment is excruciating. Why? I transfer this inner lack onto the present moment. But when I am in a state of joy? Suddenly the present moment is replete with abundance. For example, if I am stressed out about a work project, worried about how things will go, engaging in a million "what ifs," I am bound to be worn out. During this state of inner chaos, were my daughter to do something out of alignment with my expectations, it is quite possible that I would snap at her. I would project my inner misalignment onto her and our relationship. Do you see how easily this can happen? In fact, it probably happens on a daily basis for most of us.

The world we live in has conditioned us to transfer our inner discontent outwardly, either blaming others or consuming something like objects or substances. When we feel the rumblings of inner disconnect, we immediately assume something on the outside is missing. So the next time you are in the mode of finding something on the outside to blame, fix, consume, or do in order to make yourself feel happy and your life meaningful, pause and ask, What am I lacking right now? The answer will often have to do with a quest for significance. You may be seeking a particular person's validation, approval, a sense of belonging, a need for love, or a feeling of worth. This is what you are missing, not that "thing" out there.

Heal your needs by going within. As you do so, the outer quest shifts. What we thought would fulfill us loses its power. Only when we are able to pause, go within, and ask the questions I have suggested can we begin to defog our perceptions and realize that all that is missing was always within us.

You are infinitely purposeful. There is nothing you do or have done that hasn't had purpose and, therefore, profound meaning. Once you shift your perception to this new way of seeing yourself and your life, you will reframe all your experiences as pivotal to your arrival at a state of awareness. You will begin to see how all your childhood causes and effects led you to this exact moment in time.

The result is that you no longer resent or regret anything that has happened. Instead, you are humbled by their wise purpose in your awakening process and express deep gratitude for it all. The intention becomes one only—growth. Once this intention is embodied on a moment-to-moment basis, you and purpose become inseparable. Purpose breathes through you in every moment and you entwine with the aliveness of the earth around you and all its creatures.

23

Embracing Compassion

There is no compassion for another without self-compassion
There is no acceptance for another without self-acceptance
There is nothing to provide another until
we have provided for ourselves
Whatever is within will be without
It's just the inconvenient truth of being human.

I was once asked in an interview for my definition of *compassion.* I said, "self-love." The interviewer looked taken aback by my quick answer and said, "No, I mean compassion for others." I looked her square in the eyes and said, "Yes, I know. My answer is the same, self-love."

Compassion is long thought of as being for another. This belief was where I stayed stuck for many decades of my life. I didn't realize the greatest lesson of wisdom—compassion for another can only stem from compassion for the self.

Self-rejection, rather than self-love, is one of the greatest motivators of our behaviors. As long as this is true, we will engage inauthentically and dysfunctionally. Because we reject ourselves constantly, we fear this rejection from others. This keeps us searching for significance from others.

See me, see me, see me is my mantra. More specifically, *see me the way I need you to see me, so I can feel good about myself.* Little do we realize that our conciliatory behavior stems from a deeper need, even beyond the need to be loved. It comes from the need to avoid rejection.

Have you ever seen yourself become a version of yourself you barely recognize just to fit in? You begin to wear certain clothes and shoes or do your hair a certain way. Or you try hard to read certain books or watch movies just to keep up with your friends. The reason for this is self-rejection. We reject ourselves, which is why rejection by others terrifies us. It's because we cut off parts of ourselves in self-loathing in order to appear a certain way that others pick up on and cut us off. We think they are doing this, but this isn't so. We are the first to reject ourselves.

Have you ever paid attention to your inner dialogue? Have you journaled your automatic thoughts? You may be surprised. You might discover how cruel and negating your inner voice truly is. Take a pen and spill all your thoughts on the page. If you cannot think of anything at this moment, go back to a negative memory and unleash your thoughts about it. Observe how you talk about yourself and what words you use. You might be shocked at how self-scathing you are. You will be observing your lack of self-compassion.

Compassion is something we have been conditioned to believe we need to express for others, rarely thinking of meting it out to ourselves. Perhaps we associate self-compassion as arrogant, haughty, or narcissistic. Compassion has nothing to do with any of these. Compassion, at its core, has to do with a nonjudgmental understanding and acceptance of ourselves. It's easy for us to be compassionate to ourselves or others when things go our way. The real challenge is to express compassion when things don't go our way. Are you able to see the parts of yourself that are less than desirable while staying in a state of acceptance and understanding? If you are, you have achieved self-compassion.

There is no compassion for others without self-compassion. All compassion toward others starts and ends with self-compassion. If we aren't loving toward ourselves, how can we hope to be so toward others?

Integrating All Our Broken Pieces

Having compassion for ourselves means accepting all the parts of ourselves—the good, bad, and ugly. We even need to have compassion for the part of us that cannot have compassion for ourselves. We must observe all our parts as a loving mother might observe her little children, considering each of them worthy of acceptance. She doesn't just pick the tall ones or the pretty ones. She finds something endearing about all of her children because she understands how they came to be. In the same way, we too can challenge ourselves to see all parts of ourselves as worthy of understanding.

If I lost my temper with my daughter, I used to be hard on myself. I remember feeling wretched and unworthy of being a mother. I really beat myself up. I knew that this wasn't healthy for me and it was sending me down a path of more self-loathing. I lacked self-compassion for myself. When I dug deeper, I realized that I was extremely self-critical. I had placed an impossible burden of perfection on myself.

I had two parts of myself that I needed to have compassion toward—the imperfect part of me *and* the part of me that loathed imperfection. I had to love both parts. Instead of telling myself to stop being hard on myself, I began to have compassion for the side of me that felt it needed to be the matron-in-charge who needed to scold my imperfect side. My imperfect side was just being herself—fallible and human. The other part of me that wasn't letting her be imperfect was really the more tragic one, since she expected perfection.

So it is with all of us. We have this self-critical side of us that we think needs to be killed off and buried—and, indeed, she may need this. But the only way to do this is to first have compassion for why this side exists in the first place. When we show this part of ourselves understanding and care, it diminishes. This is the point of compassion—to understand all our parts, even the parts that aren't compassionate and caring.

If we are jealous of our friend and feel guilty about it, we have two parts of ourselves that need our compassion—the jealous side, and the side that reacts to this jealousy. Do you see what I mean? Sometimes, we might have three or four sides to ourselves, all demanding our understanding. Simply cutting off parts of ourselves isn't the answer. It will only further exacerbate our self-loathing. Only when we understand and integrate all parts of ourselves do we enter a state of equanimity.

This is especially true of our anxiety and anger. The more we denigrate the parts of ourselves that are prone to either, the more they grow. The only way to become less of anything is to first accept its presence. The more we resist anything, the more it grows.

You see this when you react to your children or your intimate others. If they are behaving negatively and you react to them negatively, doesn't the negative quotient grow? This is because we are fueling it with resistance rather than acceptance. The moment we see something as intelligent and natural, it no longer needs to fight for its significance. It feels acceptance and validation. Once it's seen, it doesn't need to clamor for attention and slowly fades away. Acceptance is like magic.

Entering Wholeness

Self-compassion is different from self-esteem or self-affirmation. The latter focus on being positive and thinking highly of oneself. True self-compassion is not interested in either of these. It has nothing to do with feeling good about ourselves and everything to do with simply accepting ourselves. The goal of self-compassion isn't to be more joyful or more of anything. It's simply to be one thing only—self-accepting. We don't need to see ourselves as better-than or worse-than. There is zero judgment or comparison. We should just see ourselves as we are and allow ourselves to be. Even if we are judgmental, we must see this part of us with compassion as well.

Self-esteem focuses on feeling good about ourselves and on praising our positive attributes. Self-compassion moves beyond this to where we love those parts of ourselves that aren't so praiseworthy and allow them to exist as they are—no touch-ups, no changes. This requires us to see ourselves as fully human and therefore quite ordinary. When we release the desire to be extraordinary and surrender to the messy, chaotic, and extremely fallible parts of ourselves, we embrace our full humanity. We expect nothing more of ourselves than varying degrees of imperfection.

We apply the principle of nonduality to our inner self. Rather than seeing ourselves as lacking and missing x or y, we see ourselves as whole in this moment in time, just as we are. Sure, we understand that we are works in progress, but this doesn't mean that whoever we are in this moment is incomplete. As we see ourselves through the eyes of wholeness, we begin to integrate our broken pieces into one unified circle of completion.

Our lack of courage only exists because of our fear of rejection. Once we have fully accepted ourselves, how can we experience rejection? The two cannot coexist. The only reason another can reject us is because, somewhere inside, we believe we are rejectable, and the only reason for this is because we have rejected ourselves.

If we have accepted ourselves for all our human elements and another judges us, we don't lose our equilibrium. If they call us "nasty" or "uncaring," we only have two responses: either we agree because we have already accepted that part of ourselves and moved on, or we don't agree because we know that is not who we are and move on. Either way, we don't resist the other's view of us. Their perception of us remains theirs. We don't rob the other of their right to their perception. We honor it and celebrate their freedom to hold this viewpoint.

Once we enter full acceptance of ourselves, we allow others to have any perception of us they wish. Releasing our own and another's ideas of superiority, we stay grounded in our inherent interconnectedness. No one is better than or worse than another. There is no more comparing. Each one of us is simply a human with vastly different strengths and limitations.

Wanting to be like someone else or to be liked by them is to be resistant to our diversity. Once we accept ourselves as humans who manifest a spectrum of traits, we stop wishing and wanting to possess traits we don't or can't have. We accept our height, our looks, our IQ. Where we can grow, we try to, but we do so without fighting who we naturally are.

The core quality of self-compassion is self-ease. I see self-ease as the antidote to dis-ease. When we are light, forgiving, and easy on ourselves, we flow within ourselves and allow ourselves to recover from mistakes, forgoing emotional baggage. We tell ourselves that it's okay to mess up and that we can try harder next time. Or we tell ourselves that good enough is more than enough.

When I lowered my standards of perfection to simply trying to be good enough, everything changed in my mothering. I stopped pushing myself toward unrelenting standards and, in this way, stopped pushing my daughter. As I eased myself into my humanity, I did the same for my daughter. The less I saw myself through critical eyes, the less I saw her through those eyes.

This is the magic of self-compassion. As we release ourselves into a full acceptance of our humanity, we release others. Realizing how we have inherited dysfunctional patterns of relating and loving, we accept that others have inherited such patterns as well. Just as we don't expect ourselves to let go of all negativity at one time, we don't expect others to do so either. We see ourselves in everyone else and everyone else in us. No longer are we superior or inferior to anyone.

Thich Nhat Hanh's poem "Call Me by My True Names" is a call to self-compassion. He describes himself across an array of human possibilities and qualities—for example, as both the one who is raped and the rapist. There is no separation between us as individuals. We are mirrors of each other. The thief that we judge "out there" is someone we could one day become if the circumstances for thieving arose. Similarly, the person we judge as angry or rageful "out there" is no different from someone we have been in our past or might one day be in our future. It all depends on the life circumstances that shape us all.

When parents confess to me that they lost their temper with their children and got mad at them, perhaps even slapping them, they say this in shame and expect me to judge them. When I don't, they are shocked. I explain to them that I have been them in my past, and I may be them again in my future. It's just a matter of what the circumstances are that might or might not trigger my own conditioned and limited beliefs. This level of compassion allows them to release their shame. They begin to understand themselves with the same level of understanding I mirror for them. It's here they can grow and evolve into more loving beings. If they didn't receive this level of understanding, they would stay stuck in guilt and shame, both of which obstruct growth.

Acceptance of our shadow takes infinite self-compassion. Most of us deny our shadow or rationalize it in some way. Only when we fully acknowledge its elements do we understand ourselves and others.

You may ask, "How do I have compassion for someone I don't like?" I always explain that compassion means understanding and accepting who we and others are. It doesn't mean we endorse the behaviors or even encourage them. All it means is that we understand how we and the other got to be where we are. Once we do, we have the freedom to choose whether we continue the same way or change.

Once we see the potential for all types of behaviors to exist within us, we are compassionately accepting of these possible shadow elements within and extend this kindness to others. Before rushing to judgment, we remember to pause and see ourselves in their circumstances, knowing that the only thing that separates us is our life situation. We see our underlying common humanity and forge connection with their plight rather than disconnection. This is how we raise each other up, building bridges toward each other rather than widening crevices.

All our suffering emerges from lack of acceptance of the self. If we were in touch with the whole of our human potential and compassionately accepted these elements, we would see ourselves as one with all humanity. Once we see this underlying unity, we enter a communality. Our suffering ends when we see that we are all in the same boat, each struggling with our unique insecurities. Then compassion abounds. We begin to feel another's pain more than before. Our capacity for empathy rises and our relationships become more joyful and fulfilling. It all begins and ends with our own self-compassion.

~

24

Embracing the Inner Parent

As we evolve, we forgive our parents for their humanity
We release them from our expectations and needs
We activate our own inner mothering
And reparent the wounds they left bereft and bare
And soon realize that we were our own healers all along.

I tell all my "chronologically adult" clients, those over twenty-one, that their ultimate healing will only occur once they move beyond the limits of their childhood and the parenting they received. This is a foreign concept to most of them. So entrenched are they to being their parents' children, with all the wounding that was created, that to think of themselves as moving beyond this is terrifying. Who are they if not their conditioning, their past, and the parenting they received?

I still remember feeling dejected when I noticed how my father pulled away from being "fatherly" when he retired around the age of sixty-five. I was twenty-eight at the time. He seemed to be interested in living out his retirement years on his own schedule and appeared less focused on the nitty-gritty details of my life. It was like he was "done" with being a father. At first I wanted to sulk. I wanted to throw a tantrum as I watched him pull away. I took it personally. However, after sitting with my feelings for around ten days, I came to a new realization. What if he was done with his role as a father? What would that mean for me? Why would that be such a bad thing? Was it possible for us to move into an expanded awareness as good friends?

I was already living my own life in the United States and rarely saw him. I probed deeper into the fear that emerged. It wasn't as if he wasn't present for me or loving, he was just less involved than I was used to. I asked myself why I needed my father to stay exactly the same as I had known him, and why I couldn't release him to be whoever he wished now that I was a full-fledged adult. It couldn't be that I wasn't loved, because I felt very loved by him. It couldn't be that I wasn't validated or worthy, because he made me feel these things consistently. So what was it? Ah, the answer was suddenly clear. I was afraid to grow up and stop relying on him as my "daddy."

I just wasn't ready to be an adult, fully on my own. In retrospect, I can see how my father was ahead of the game. He recognized the adult in me and saw that I was ready to fly on my own. He pulled back, not out of lack of love or commitment but out of realism. Instead of inserting himself where there was no real need, he wisely discerned that his time in the forefront of my life had passed. He could now focus on other things. In his own way, he was passing the baton of my care to me. It's just that I wasn't ready to take the lead and fly, but it was precisely what I needed at the time.

Releasing Our Parents

As children, we often don't recognize that our parents are human, fallible, and ordinary—at times even fumbling and messed up. We have this fantasy that they are omniscient and omnipotent. Around our teens, the veneer of perfection gets chipped away. We catch glimpses of their ordinary humanness. Typically, we get turned off and withdraw somewhat, moving toward our peers. However, we still hold them to the expectation that they will always be there for us. If they aren't, we give ourselves the right to feel hurt and disappointed.

I have some clients in their sixties who are still tied to the umbilical cord. Fully enmeshed with their parents, they are deeply ensconced in the roles they have been playing since childhood. If the child never really adults up, neither parent nor child lets go and both have the power to trigger each other.

The fact is, most of us don't really want to grow up. So accustomed are we to the codependent relationship we share with our parents that we cannot fathom our identity away from them. In their eyes, we never grow up and, in our eyes, we don't have to. This stagnation is not only dysfunctional but also unhealthy for both the child and parent.

As long as we rely on our parents' auspices for comfort, protection, and care in adulthood, we will never activate our own capacity for these abilities within ourselves. Not only will we stagnate, we will overtax our aging parents and obstruct them from entering a new phase of their lives.

Detachment from our parents is not cold or selfish. As I already discussed, it's often the most important thing we need to do in order to enjoy a healthy individuation. Especially in the case of parent-child relationships, at some point both need to release the other to live autonomously and freely. Whether the child in the dynamic wants it or not, at some point the adult needs to stop feeding it from the breast. Children need to grow up and walk on their own for their ultimate emotional health.

What if we gave our parents an expiration date for parenting and released them from their roles after we turned a certain age? What if we gave them the freedom to choose how they wished to parent after a certain amount of time in our adulthood?

Once I released my fears around growing up, I was able to tell both my parents, "You are now released from having to take care of me. You have done enough. You have earned the right to retire from parenthood. It's not a life sentence. You are free to be. It's now my time to be my own parent." Of course, my mother took this to mean the end of my need for her and cried, but my father understood. He nodded and said with a chuckle, "Yes, you don't need me anymore in that same way. I am always here as your friend. If anything, you can take care of me now."

To allow our parents to retire from their job because we are now ready to take the helm of our own growth is a tremendous gift. It's both a release of the apron strings and a passing of the baton. It's up to both the parents and the child to execute this transformation. Through this encounter, a true coming together of spirits becomes possible.

Releasing the Past

As we release our parents from being parents, we also release them for their past culpabilities. This is not an easy thing to do, especially if one experienced a traumatic childhood. It's understandable that there may be resentment and unprocessed pain.

There are many clients I know that cannot stop the parental blame game. They cannot let all that past hurt dissolve. If you are someone for whom this rings true, I want you to know I understand. If your childhood was robbed from you due to another's unconsciousness, you likely feel resentful and angry. This is normal. However, this is what I need you to know: The longer you stay stuck in resentment toward your parents, or anyone for that matter, the longer you stay dependent on them. You are emotionally married to them.

At some point in our adult life, the rubber meets the road and we need to decide how long we are going to carry the axe from our past. When will we release our parents from their unconscious part? When will we start taking responsibility for our present?

When we decide to release our parents from their past culpability in our childhood, we do so with a compassionate understanding of their humanity and of their inevitable limitations. We see them for who they are versus through the child lenses we have been wearing. We may see extreme flaws or inadequacies that we want to turn away from. This is natural. But along the way, what we may also see is their extreme inner pain. When we touch this pain within them and have empathy for their own childhoods, we will finally be able to see them as more than just our parents. We will see them for their past and their place in a grand lineage of pain and joy. We may, for the first time, understand how generational patterns run through families and realize our power to disrupt the ones that emerge out of unconsciousness.

Instead of begrudging the childhood we had or the relationships we shared with them thus far, we see the flaws as gifts that have helped us become who we are today. We realize that every childhood has its own issues, and we release our fantasy that ours should have been different. We allow our past to stay in the past and begin to take charge of our destiny in the present.

We may believe that the release of our parents is for them. We couldn't be more wrong. It's more for us than it could ever be for them. Only when we can release them fully are we free to do what we needed to do all along, the inner work of growing up.

Becoming Our Own Parent

Releasing our parents is a huge step toward emotional liberation. But this is only the first step. After this comes the real work—stepping into the role they didn't fully complete. We need to reparent ourselves. But now we do so from the point of view of an *adult*.

Reading these pages is part of your reparenting process. By looking at yourself and doing your own inner work, you are releasing your parents of the responsibility of your emotional growth and taking yourself in your own charge. This is the pathway of truly "adulting"—from little girl to awakened woman.

Reparenting is the key to our spiritual and emotional expansion. It means we start to address those parts of ourselves that grew up with the false idea that we were not worthy, valid, or significant. We heal the "little child" within us by recognizing this "child" is only an echo of voices from our past, not who we are as an adult today. She is a phantom based on our past life.

How does this "little child" show up? It shows up in the ways we speak to ourselves, *the inauthentic voices in our mind*. We all have voices within. Some have benevolent voices and others harsh critics. One of my colleagues, Ellie, used to call her inner voices "a tribunal of assholes." These inner voices are those internalized by our inner child when we were growing up. They feel so real that we think they are our authentic voice. Some of the voices require that we hear them and soothe them. Others require a swift time out, and yet others require that we ignore them. Depending on the quality of the voice, a different reparenting strategy is required. Just like a parent is different with each child, so it is here. We need to pay attention to the inner voice and treat it with the most attuned parenting approach possible. One size doesn't fit all.

How to do this is best illustrated by what happened to one of my dearest friends, Alexa. She was describing her mental anguish and the way she constantly felt rejected and unworthy. The reason Alexa felt this way is because she *believed* the voices in her mind. I asked her to give me a play-by-play of the voices. She immediately began to choke up and cry. "I feel embarrassed to share this with you," she said. But then she continued, "You are so stupid and ugly. You aren't good at anything you do. Why would anyone want to be with you? You are just totally messed up." When I asked her to tell me who these voices reminded her of, she immediately said, "My father."

Do you see the point I am making? Those voices weren't her true self—they were voices she internalized from her father.

Although Alexa was aware that she had greatly suffered at the hands of her abusive alcoholic father, she hadn't quite seen how she had internalized his voice and was far more abusive to herself than he had ever been. Until that moment, she had just presumed these voices were her own. She was shocked when I asked her to consider that *she had actually become her own cruel father*. Her real father didn't come close to her own inner interpretation of the toxic ideas she had bought into.

Between her tears, she described feeling attacked by her inner voices. I asked her to label them. She said, "They're like cockroaches inside me, crawling all over, spreading germs. I just want to run away from my mind and my life. I never want to get up because each day they are still there. I want to die."

I encouraged her to face the cockroaches and start exterminating them—not by arguing with them, but by taking a hose of consciousness and spraying them into oblivion. For this to occur, she would first need to meet each voice head-on, naming it and *then seeing it as part of her unconsciousness*. She would need to see it as a representation of her abusive father and dissociate from such voices. *Only then would she be able to separate the cockroaches from who she is intrinsically in the present moment and see them as vestiges of her past.*

Alexa resisted me, saying that the last thing she wanted to do was confront her childhood fears. She said she had spent her whole life running away from them. I showed her that she might have avoided her past, but the fact that she lived in daily anguish showed that she could never fully run away. It was time for Alexa to face her past and address the wounds within.

We can't run away from our past. It is only through a bold confrontation of our wounds that we begin to heal what was left unhealed. It takes great courage to reimagine a new sense of self. No longer stuck in fear, passivity, servile compliance, or blame, we realize that in order to change our tomorrow, we need to refashion every single piece of who we are today.

The place to begin this journey is in our mind. What are my thoughts about myself and my world? Where did these thoughts come from? Whose voices do I play out in my mind? Are these my voices or my culture's? How can I fashion a new inner script so I can live my highest potential? Voice by voice, lie by lie, we begin the process of undoing our unconscious past. In doing so, we consciously build a new way of being.

If there is hurt from some long-ago wound, the way forward is to recognize that our core self, our essence, was never affected by this hurt. Only an aspect of our ego was wounded, not who we really are at our core. Our true self can never be wounded, only prevented from growing in the way it should. The task of reparenting is to spot those areas where we are still coming from a childish pattern of behavior that, due to our particular family's situation, did not facilitate the development of our true self in some areas of our life.

Growing ourselves up means acknowledging the circumstances in which we act in a childish manner. Activating our parent is a crucial piece of growing up. We embody the voice and being-state of the parent we may never had had in real life—the parent that sees us, soothes us, and allows us a safe space to express our truth.

If we feel anxious, instead of dealing with it through numbing ourselves or reacting outwardly, our inner parent steps in and counsels us. She might inquire, What is this anxiety about? What is triggering you? How can I support you and help you get your needs met? She activates a dialogue with the wounded parts of our inner self and allows space for the voice to speak. The anxious part of us might say, "I'm afraid that I'm not good enough and that I will be rejected in some way." The inner parent then uncovers the reasons for this and might ask, "What old memory is being triggered right now to make you feel this way? What story are you replaying right now?" The childish pattern might reply, "I remember my mother telling me I was stupid and that I should never speak up in public."

In this way, back and forth, our inner parent listens to the plaintive cries of the past and tries to uncover the real reason behind the current feelings. Like a good therapist or wise sage, the inner parent helps the childlike part of us calm down and enter a sense of worth and belonging. This part of us feels heard and understood, which results in immediate insight and relief. Rather than blindly acting out through an emotional reaction, inner dialogue allows time to pause and reflect. Through these constant validations of our essential self, the parts of us stuck in childish behavior come out of the shadows and enter a state of wholeness. In this way, our old wounds, left abandoned in childhood, get a chance to heal. No longer do we feel the need to split off these old parts of ourselves, for we see that they are *just projections from our past.*

Our projections, expectations, and relationships soon no longer reflect dysfunctional and toxic patterns from an unconscious upbringing. As our essence comes fully into being, our external relationships also fall into alignment with our inherent wholeness.

Reparenting ourselves is our way of taking personal responsibility for our own growth and healing. It's our gift to ourselves. By continually asking, What do I need right now? and, What can I offer myself right now? we activate our own inner resources to heal what was left wounded way back when.

If we don't step into the role of parenting ourselves, we will forage the earth for that mom or dad "out there." This is what most relationships act out on some level—each in the couple looking for their missing parent in the other. When we put the onus on the other to be our missing parent, things go drastically awry. Few adults are equipped with the psychological skills to provide this for the other, and it isn't their job anyway.

When thrust into this role by the other, resentment brews. Many women complain that they end up in relationships where they feel as if they are their partner's mother. No one wants to feel burdened with this responsibility. If a woman does happen to take this on her shoulders, she ends up enabling the other in unhealthy ways, mothering the other in ways that prevent them from growing.

Reparenting ourselves involves giving ourselves the tools and skills we didn't receive from our own parents to help us manage our inner world. It involves building an inner emotional toolkit filled with words that can help us find our worth and power. Our inner parent might say things like this when the time appears:

I see you, I hear you, I validate you.
You are good enough as you are.
You don't need to be perfect.
It's okay to feel this way. All your feelings are valid.
You are powerful beyond description, and you can do this.
You are capable and worthy.
You deserve to speak your will and your voice.
Your expression is important.
What happened in your childhood wasn't your fault.

Don't be afraid to create a boundary for yourself.
It is time to accept who you are without apology.

Our inner parent is our greatest advocate and coach, sometimes soft on us and yet, at other times, challenging us in ways that make us uncomfortable. Just as we need our real parents to soothe us at times but also to create boundaries, we begin to give these things to ourselves.

Reparenting involves overriding our old conditioning and developing a healthier way of being. This requires that we be brave enough to look in the mirror and truly acknowledge our unhealthy patterns, calling on our inner courage to disrupt such patterns with ways that suit our present situation.

I grew up with an extremely empathic mother who was undyingly present and loving. However, because of her own conditioning, she didn't teach me the valuable skill of laying down boundaries. She was afraid of conflict and dealt with her discomfort by pleasing people to the point of utter self-abnegation. I learned to be the same way through osmosis. As a result, I entered many relationships where I departed from my true self in order to keep the peace and harmony.

As a result, I martyred myself, and then eventually grew bitter and resentful because I allowed myself to be constantly violated. My lack of boundaries was showing up everywhere, especially in my work, where I was unable to create clear perimeters around people's demands of my presence and time. As a result, I was overworked. I had to emotionally straightjacket myself so that I didn't overdo, over-give, and overcommit. I had to learn to say things like, "I will get back to you," or "I have to think about it." I had to create new neural pathways so that reactions wouldn't pop out of my mouth without a pause. I had to undo all my instinctual ways of responding and replace them with more conscious ones. Most of all, I had to learn to love and honor myself. I had to become my own parent.

This process speaks to the emotional and spiritual reparenting that is essential if we are to fully heal ourselves. I now needed to teach myself what my mother couldn't. My first step was to release her of any blame or responsibility. I couldn't keep blaming my childhood for my abysmal lack of boundaries. I needed to show up for myself. I began to read up on the patterns of the classic empath and how we unconsciously enter codependent and abusive relationships. I began to deconstruct my patterns and notice how I set up dynamics that were primed for boundary violations.

It was shocking to see how my one childhood pattern kept recreating itself, wounding me over and over. I entered a state of compassion for my mother and for how she had abnegated herself because of never learning this skill in her own childhood. I was able to trace this pattern to my grandmother, my mother's mother, and began to see how the dominoes tumbled through the generations. It was now on me to disrupt my matrilineal pattern. Would I be able to show up for myself and learn this valuable skill and, through this, teach my daughter what I had never learned?

Piece by piece, chain by chain, I began undoing my patterns of blind empathy. I began to see how my people-pleasing was really people-fearing stemming from a lack of self-worth. I knew I needed to give myself the empowerment and self-love to stand up for myself in a way my mother couldn't teach me. It was terrifying at first. So conditioned was I to fear rejection and conflict that I instinctively bowed down and cowered instead of stepping into my voice.

Each time I noticed my pattern, I soothed my fears and gently challenged myself to be brave. Each time I spoke up just a little more, and then a little more. Each time I experienced my greatest fear, which was rejection. Instead of capitulating to old patterns, I kept practicing using my voice and creating boundaries in my relationships. I began to say "no" and "no more" consistently and vociferously.

Although terrified, I stepped away from relationships that locked me in old patterns. I became comfortable losing people and stepped into the discomfort of being alone. Because I had my inner parent there by my side, I was able to trust my own company more. I began relying on others less to give me my sense of validation and was able to honor my own voice and ways more.

Reparenting ourselves involves creating and relying on our

inner GPS. Instead of looking outward toward others to mother, father, and guide us, we activate these powerful elements within ourselves. Just as a parent encourages the toddler to learn to walk step-by-step, here too we gently cajole ourselves to act autonomously. Each time we enter self-doubt and believe we don't have our own answers, we halt in our tracks and say, "There is no one out there who knows me more than I do. I have the answers within me. Look inside and I will find them."

As we practice self-reliance, our inner GPS becomes honed. It speaks to us in louder voices because we have finally emboldened it through our self-trust. Our inner radar turns within at every turn, taking us closer and closer to our truth until we finally arrive at our greatest gift and destination: self-honor and governance.

The Healer Within

There is a famous Zen saying, "If you meet the Buddha on the road, kill him." What this profound statement means is that the Buddha, or the enlightened one, can never be found on the outside, only within ourselves. As long as we believe that we are lesser-than another, we will never reach our true potential.

The word *kill* is used to jolt us into the power of a spiritual warrior who is adept at demolishing illusions. The task here is to "kill" our false idea that we are followers rather than leaders. As long as we are attached to another as our leader, we will stray. After all, the most wise leaders are those who lead us back to our own wisdom, for they know that each of us is capable of finding exactly what we need within our own being.

We are each on a journey, walking on our own path. Staying in our own lane and seeing the beauty of the scenery—be it flowers or thorny shrubs—along our path is the way of wisdom. Straying from this path to follow another's path is the way of delusion.

On a more profound level, this saying reminds us of the interconnectedness of all beings. There is no one on the outside that doesn't exist on the inside. What we recognize in another has to first exist in ourselves, so the fact that we see wisdom within another means that this wisdom also has to exist within us. The other is simply a mirror. Understanding this on a deeply spiritual level allows us to liberate ourselves from our tethers of dependency on another—be it a parent, our children, our partners, or our teachers.

As a person who people describe as "a teacher," I see how easy it is for others to project their insecurities onto me. In a myriad of ways, I receive all sorts of labels and judgments. Sometimes I am placed by another in the role of neglectful mother where, without my awareness, I am seen as critical and abandoning. They might also put me in the role of loving mother, where they see me as magnanimous and nurturing. Or they might put me on a pedestal as a wise sage who has all the solutions and answers.

At first, I felt I needed to prove myself to others. At other times, I felt resentful and victimized. As I did my own inner work and came into my inner knowing, I began to understand that these projections onto me were reflections of the others' broken pieces and had little or nothing to do with me.

Once I understood this, I stopped having negative reactions toward these people and began harboring compassion toward them. I was able to separate my knowledge and trust in myself from who they needed me to be for their own spiritual growth. Of course, this could only come about after I saw how I too did the same to others. It was only when I "killed the Buddha" in my own life that I understood this process more deeply and compassionately.

There is another Buddhist teaching that asks us to look at all sentient beings as our own mother. What this means again is to see everyone on the outside as a reflection of ourselves. No one is separate from us. We are all interconnected and one. When we deeply understand this, we cut through the illusion of believing that someone on the outside can fulfill our inner emotional needs. We realize that this external person we are searching for is really the one who lives within us. We are that salve, salvation, guru, and healer. That is us and we are that.

~

25

Embracing Detachment

Am I a loving person or just attached?
This is the ultimate question we each need to answer
Attachment is always needy, conditional, and dependent
It keeps us tethered, weighted, bound, and gagged
True love does the opposite. It powers our wings to fly free.

One of the most shocking realizations arrived for me when I became aware that most of my relationships were based on attachment, not love. Up until that moment, I had fully believed that I had loved many and been loved by many. This awareness shook me to my core. I had so identified with the idea that I was a loving person. To understand that this love was laced with attachment was unnerving.

As a spiritual warrior, I was aware that I needed to observe my shadow elements, the parts I didn't want to look at. I needed to push myself to new frontiers so that I could enter higher states of consciousness around my actions and hidden agendas. Understanding the fundamental difference between attachment and love catapulted my spiritual growth and relationships to another level. Perhaps this can be an invitation for you to evolve in a similar way as well.

The Nature of Life

We attach to things, time, events, people, places, ideas, and most of all the *idea* of attachment. We attach because we don't understand that the fundamental quality of the nature of life, as the Buddha so eloquently taught, is impermanence.

All that exists is impermanent. Nothing lasts. The only constant is change. When we don't fully appreciate this simple but profound truth, we suffer. Impermanence means everything is transient and therefore is bound to be lost to us in some way, shape, or form. To love and honor life is to love and honor its impermanence.

All things are rising and fading in the moment—right here, right now. The present moment is all we have, but as soon as it arrives, we lose it and it disappears. Such awareness of the utter moment-by-moment nature of life allows us to stay nonattached. Instead of attaching, we enter the presence I talked about earlier where we enliven each moment by being fully attuned and attentive. In this way, we appreciate every moment for what it brings us and don't cling to it when it passes.

When we attach to something or some idea, we believe we then exist in connection to it. This "thing" gives us significance and validity. But if we understood that this significance and validation is in itself an illusion, as it can never come from the outside, then we can be nonattached. So, in essence, whatever it is we are craving is an illusion.

This is a hard concept to live by, especially when we have been conditioned to live the opposite way by clinging, craving, attaching, and possessing. However, when we understand how this conditioned way has brought us so much suffering, we may be willing to let it go. Attachment will always bring about suffering because we are going to lose this thing sooner or later. So when we attach, we need to realize that we are setting ourselves up for suffering. When we suffer from losing x, y, or z, we fall prey to the false idea that x, y, or z has "left" us or that we have "lost." In essence, none of this has happened. After all, can we really lose something that was never ours to begin with? When we understand this, we connect to things, places, people, and ideas with the right frame of mind. We understand that this connection is in the here and now only.

This doesn't mean our connection to another isn't vital or strong.

It is. But it needs to be indelibly tempered with nonattachment. This practice of nonattachment is called *detachment*. It's one of the more abstract concepts of spirituality that we need to grasp if we are to evolve as liberated individuals. It's pivotal.

When my daughter was born, I named her Maia, meaning *illusion*. The reason I did so was to remind myself that my attachment to her is an illusion and that she is her own free spirit. When I see her as "my" daughter, I immediately set myself up for possession and control. The identification that she is mine becomes fixed and rigid. With this come all sorts of expectations and ownership, as if she is a thing to be had that I can hold on to. This is the way most parents treat their children. In this way, we set both our children and ourselves up for suffering.

Instead, when I release my daughter from my ownership, I see her as a being that came through me. I see her as part of all life in the universe, and, as such, not belonging to me alone. This latter perspective allows me to detach from my desire to control her and release her to live the life she needs to live in order to thrive.

When we appreciate the impermanent nature of life, we appreciate the joy of life. After all, if my biology was permanent and fixed, I would not have been able to conceive my daughter. We need impermanence in life. Without it, life wouldn't be life. It would be death. If the caterpillar wasn't impermanent, there wouldn't be any butterflies. Similarly, we wouldn't be here today. We would still be infants. Do you see how impermanence is the very force of life that allows us to keep living?

Knowing That We Don't Know

For those who meditate, the concept of impermanence is amply clear. We come to realize that what we once believed was a solid body and a solid mind is not that at all. We begin to see that our body is made up of innumerable pulsating sensations. So too our minds are made up of innumerable thoughts that keep pulsating. It is here we are given the first glimpse into our identity. In essence, we are just a conglomeration of sensations and thoughts, rising and falling, moment after moment. There is no such thing as a fixed body or mind. They are always in flux and flow, constantly transforming.

The realization that our thoughts are impermanent can at first be disorienting, but it soon comes to be reassuring. On the one hand, we may feel unsettled realizing that our thoughts are never "real" in that they never stay constant. But, on the other hand, we may come to see that since they never stay constant anyway, we can choose which ones to think about and which ones to discard. In other words, we may come to see that we are not enslaved by our thoughts.

Our thoughts are not "insane." They are just impermanent. So it is with every cell in our body. All of nature is constantly on the move. When our child has a change of mood and throws a tantrum, we suffer. When the economy collapses and we lose our job, we suffer. When our lover abandons us and leaves us, we suffer. The fundamental cause of our suffering? Our false delusion that none of this *should* happen. But this is exactly what should happen as per the nature of life. Things are supposed to rise and fall, like the breath in our chest, every single moment. No two moments are supposed to be alike. Nothing is the same, ever. Things are constantly changing, moment after moment after moment.

You see, this idea that things, as well as our bodies, are living and dying every single moment is a highly uncomfortable one. It is one that we simply cannot tolerate. It brings about too much anxiety. It doesn't allow us to create a fixed idea of who and what we are. It doesn't allow us to rest in a known future. We realize now that because things are constantly changing, it's impossible to predict or control the future. This is a hard reality to face. In our ignorance, we desire to know our future.

It's our human nature to want to know things. After all, if things are constantly changing, then what's going to happen next? And more importantly, who will we be tomorrow? And in the next moment?

With this awareness and acceptance of the unknown comes pain, of course. It is hard to let go of our desire for control and constancy. Pain is a natural part of life and our growing awareness. We cannot resist it. We are going to lose things and people we love. We are going to age, and so on. And most importantly, we are always going to be unable to predict the future, even though we most desperately want to.

The wise know they have arrived at wisdom when they can say, "I know that I don't know." They have released their attachment to certainty and predictability. They have accepted that the reason they suffer is because they are attached to things they cannot control. They have let go of this attachment. When we recognize the truth that all we know is that everything changes and, therefore, we cannot know it all, we arrive at a place of higher spiritual evolution.

Entering a space of "I don't know" is to enter the abundant mystery of the universe. It's to stay grounded in the groundlessness of things. Here we don't seek to make up fantastical stories about creation or destruction. We don't seek to know what is essentially unknowable. We allow for the unknown to be exactly that—unknown. Instead of egoically trying to impose an answer on an unanswerable reality, we wisely release this craving and, instead, cultivate the art of knowing what we do know—the awareness of the present moment.

What Healthy Detachment Means in Practice

I have covered this topic all through this book because it is such an important one, for us women especially. I am circling back in this section to make things crisper and clearer for you. I am trying to embed these core principles within your psyche so you can implement them with ease and comfort.

It's important not to confuse attachment with Attachment Parenting, a school of parenting that fosters a deep connection between parent and child. Attachment in Attachment Parenting is beneficial and is the foundation of a healthy bond between parent and child. The way I use the term *attachment* is more in the Buddhist sense, where it is not about connection and bonding, but about an unhealthy entanglement, dependency, and borderline addiction.

When we think of the words *nonattachment* or *detachment*, we may immediately associate them with coldheartedness or indifference—as if we are being aloof, closed off, and distant, as well as selfish and self-absorbed. Detachment is actually the opposite. What it really means is that because we so understand that impermanence is a vital aspect of all of life, we release all false clinging. We enter what is known as a "letting go." This letting go, or surrender, implies an unequivocal acceptance of the fundamental reality of life *as-is*.

This dissolution of expectations allows us to enter unconditional love. It's in this state of awareness that we become more loving and more connected, warm, and nurturing. Consider these statements:

A grandmother tells her grandson, "I never want you to become an artist like your father. You must do something better with your life."
A fathers tells his daughter, "I don't want you to cut your hair because you will look like a boy and it won't suit you."
A friend tells another, "I really need you to stop speaking to your neighbor because I don't like her."
A wife tells her husband, "I want you to fire your secretary because she makes me uncomfortable."
A husband tells his wife, "I don't want you to go on your girls' trip because they drink and I don't like that."

Each of these individuals will claim that they love the other and are actually saying these things out of care and concern for their well-being. But are they really? Are they caring about the other or about themselves? Can you see how attached they are to their own point of view, their own expectations, and their own desires? When we don't examine how our identities are attached to the other, we can impose ourselves on the other without even consciously realizing it. In these ways, our caring doesn't feel like caring at all.

One of the greatest gifts we can bequeath to another is to recognize when our love turns to attachment. We notice when we begin to "use" the other for our fulfillment and cling to them for validation. Or we notice how we project our needs and expectations onto them. This awareness allows us to shift from projection to introspection. As we turn inward, we pay attention to the patterns we are playing out. We absolve the other from holding the responsibility of filling us up and validating us.

Detachment doesn't mean we avoid becoming intimate with the other, only that we aren't dependent on them for our inner nourishment. We receive the other's love and care as they choose to share it, without judging or critiquing its form. We move away from small-minded concerns such as, Do they love me, do they desire me, do they need me? to big-minded ones such as, Are we thriving, growing, evolving, allowing, and freeing?

We move away from our fantasies of the other to an acceptance of who they truly are, shadow and all. Do you see the difference? One is about possession and control, where we try to change the other to fit our ideal. The other is about liberation and elevation, where we accept the other by helping them stay true to who they are.

Attachment tries to "fix" the other in an attempt to make them who we need them to be so we can feel whole. If they cannot or will not comply, we try to force them to do so. The other either resists or capitulates. Either way, they are inauthentic to their true nature and this will show up in other parts of the relationship. Soon, both will firmly plant themselves in their false self and relate to each other from a place of need, dependency, and control.

We are attached to our way of thinking, feeling, or opining, which includes all the things we believe are right. It's a "my way or the highway" approach. So attached are we to our way that we superimpose this on the other and become deeply attached to getting them to change.

When a person doesn't change as we would like them to, our love becomes conditional. We show our disapproval. When they acquiesce, we express praise and affirm them. It all depends on how closely or not the other matches our fantasy. As such, we are consistently prey to the other's moods and emotional well-being.

Detachment from another person or a thing only begins with a serious acknowledgment of our inner sense of lack. We are unaccustomed to viewing ourselves as autonomous emotional beings. So wedded are our emotions to elements outside of us, we are unable to break free. When the other's state is up, we are up. When they are down, we are down.

Detachment scares us because it truly demarcates us as solo beings who are walking on individual paths. The journey feels lonely and can at times be terrifying. Instead of seeing this as empowering, culture has rendered us needy. The thought of feeling full without the other feels strange. Shaking ourselves free from our dependency is the hallmark of what it means to become an adult.

The Power of Surrender

Why do relationships drain us? Is it because of the relationship, per se, or because of our mindset? In my experience, it's the latter. It all comes down to attachment. We expend so much energy on fixing and controlling the other's behavior and emotional states that we exhaust ourselves and experience disenfranchisement and eventual burnout.

The moment we release ourselves from the idea that we are in control of the other and surrender to the is-ness of the relationship, we expand ourselves exponentially. We have endless energy now to make creative choices. No longer entangled with the other's state of being, we are free to move toward paths that work best for our highest self.

By allowing individuals to unfold exactly the way they are, without conditions of control and judgment, we actually show them the greatest care and concern. While we are conditioned to associate passion with control, we now see that the greatest passion for another comes with the least control over them. So passionately in love are we with their essence that we have no desire to control them. Transcendent passion for another implies absolute relinquishment of control.

Do we love another for their essence? It's rare that we love another for their true inner being. Wrapped up and blinded by the external form, such as how a person looks and behaves, we fail to tune into the essence of their being.

Parents especially, fall into the trap of defining their love for their children according to the form of things, such as how well they achieve in school or in athletics, how popular they are, and even how happy they appear. In doing so we miss the point and fail to tune into our children's abundant and natural essence. This is why many children feel unseen, invalidated, and unloved by their parents.

Despite their parents' protests, many of my clients vehemently insist they never felt unconditional love. No matter what the parent claims, children often hold on to this view. The reason for this? The parent was caught up in attachment, where the child's *doing* was valued more than their *being*, their essence.

With our intimate partner, we make lists of the criteria they should meet. While this can be helpful on a practical level, it can never be a long-lasting strategy for a fulfilling relationship. It's almost always based on form-based aspects of a person and rarely on their essential being. As long as we focus on the form of things as opposed to their essence, we will stay mired in attachment.

When we have lots of inner holes akin to Swiss cheese, we will be on the lookout for external elements to fill these holes. These holes persist because we haven't yet entered unequivocal acceptance of ourselves in our as-is state.

Our inner "hole-ness" is what we project onto the other, which results in our trying to get them to fill our voids. We don't see ourselves as emotional predators, but we are. Just as we are predators, we are also prey for the other's predatory ways as they seek to fill their own holes. As such, we never arrive at a state of transcendent love and remain stuck at the level of attachment. Only when our inner "hole-ness" moves into inner "w"holeness can we release our attachment and surrender to transcendent love.

Detachment requires the act of graceful surrender. We don't give up the desire to be happy or joyful, but we do release the need for it to come wrapped in a particular package. Once we surrender to living life as it is, not as we believe it should be, we release others from being a certain way in order to provide for our happiness. Instead of craving happiness, we move into a state of growth by stretching ourselves to accept what is.

The Wisdom of Nonduality

With life comes death. With day comes night. With dark comes light. With yin comes yang. What these speak to is the inextricable nature of nonduality. Everything is nondual, yet we live as if everything is dual.

Because we desire to know and control our present and our future, we label things with finite categories: this and that, tall and short, fat and thin, beautiful and ugly, me and you, black and white. By dichotomizing our reality, we give ourselves the illusion of order and control.

Wisdom means to understand the nondual nature of life. There are no separate entities and everything is interconnected as one. When we become attached to ideas or "things," we separate and divide them. It's natural, isn't it?

Because we have all grown up in a conditioned world of duality, we see ourselves through the lenses of good and bad. This is a trap designed to keep us from entering a transcendent state of divinity. Paraphrasing Rumi, "Beyond our ideas of wrongdoing and right-doing, there is a field. I will meet you there." Only when we move beyond duality are we able to release our shame and enter self-love.

One of our most potent self-realizations occurs when we see how we hold the potential for all layers of good and bad. We welcome this as our human destiny. Instead of seeing ourselves as only one or the other, we embrace the potential for both.

Once we see this capacity within ourselves, we see it within others as well. Instead of holding ourselves as special, we now realize we aren't. We are different, even unique, but not special. This is a powerful spiritual awareness that allows us to enter the space of a shared humanity and, thereby, a new earth.

Moving past our individual egos, we release our egoic righteousness and judgment of ourselves or others. We understand our shared struggles and our common duress. When we see ourselves as mirrors of each other, we realize that what separates us is not some grand wisdom or intelligence but simply a confluence of life circumstances. Were we in the other person's shoes, living in their circumstance, we too might have behaved exactly as they have, doing the same things we condemn. We can only realize this when we honor our own capacity for negative behavior and fully accept our own shadow.

Understanding nonduality allows us to enter a space of nonjudgment. Here all ideas of how things "should" be get suspended. Everything exists in context and relationship to something else. More than anything, we understand that to parse and divide our reality comes from our ignorance of the true nature of things.

Everything is whole within itself. What this means is that every idea and concept holds its opposing reality within it. Hence the yin and yang symbol interweaving to form a unified whole. When we open our minds to the possibility that everything exists within everything, we stop trying to control, label, and categorize. This immediately eliminates judgment, which is the scourge of humanity.

Surrendering to nonduality allows us to enter a state of allowance. There is no one way things or people should be. There is no such thing as perfection, failure, success, or good or bad. This allows the people in our lives to be flawed and fallible. The more we enter our own inner wholeness, the more we enter self-acceptance. Self-acceptance automatically translates to acceptance of all others.

Part of self-acceptance involves letting go of perfection as a goal. We see its illusory nature. Once we do, we fully embrace the other in their totality, including their strengths and their failings. Just as we don't bemoan the rose for its thorns, we don't judge the other for their failings. The moment we surrender to this mindset, our suffering radically reduces. We not only free ourselves of judgment of how things "should" be, we release others to be exactly who they are. Surrendering judgment allows us to be free. Those around us also experience this freedom. Love becomes synonymous with freedom. Ultimately, freedom is the only goal of love.

Transcendent love involves care for all, whether or not they meet our expectations. The other is not seen through the lens of whether they are utilitarian, but instead they are only seen for their essence. As such, they are celebrated as our teachers. Because every human being is our teacher, we celebrate all who enter our life. Our love for the teachings they mete out stays constant as there are always lessons to learn. How can we turn against our teacher? Only when we turn against the teaching do we enter a state of blame toward the individual. However, if we see every teaching as valuable, we then value every teacher. This is how we move beyond conditionality and enter a state of unconditional love.

26

Embracing Emptiness

I thought I knew who I was
Certain of my names and titles
Certain of my roles and labels
Certain of my past and future
Oh, what a mirage all this is.

We are not who we think we are. Who we think we are is a conditioned version of ourselves that we have been acting out since we were born. Before we even leave our mother's womb, we are already stamped with a zillion identities—our family name and traditions, our religion and its accompanying God and beliefs, culture's educational values and pressures, beliefs around race, success, achievement, beauty, sexuality, worth, and society. We basically inherit our parents' consciousness or lack thereof. There is no escaping this transfer of conditioning. It happens involuntarily most of the time. None of this is who we truly are.

When we are unconscious and unawakened, we allow our mind to be left unexplored and unexamined. We are fully asleep. We look awake, but we are, in effect, asleep. We remain captive to the past and all the cultural identifications that go with it. Too often, we proceed to make our children our captives as well. So the legacies are passed on, generation to generation.

As I have mentioned throughout this book, to "wake up" means to demolish our attachments and break free of our mental cages.

We wake up to the fact that we have been brainwashed. Now it is time to rid ourselves of all the mental garbage we have been steeped in. This process of awakening is a process of emptying the mind of its unconsciousness and therefore toxic beliefs. As we free ourselves, we empty the container that carries all these false identifications and begin to touch upon our true nature.

The Misbeliefs About Beliefs

Our beliefs about life and people shape our every moment. The more we believe, the more we are contoured by these beliefs. The more strongly we adhere to these beliefs, the more rigidly attached we are to them and the more zealous we are to stay in accordance with them. How can we expect to live a life of freedom and spontaneity when these beliefs shutter us behind their bars?

Our beliefs about life stop us from fully living. Because we haven't even woken up to the fact that our beliefs are inherited by osmosis from our childhoods and culture, we think that what we believe is who we are. There is no separation between our beliefs and our identity. Our beliefs *are* our identity. Many fundamentalists die for their beliefs because their life *is* their beliefs. Their beliefs have taken over and dictate their identity, so much so that their identity and their beliefs are one and the same.

For example, if we inherited a belief system from our past that we are lazy, and this was deeply entrenched within us, imagine how it would color the reality of our experiences and our relationships. Every time we felt neglected by another, it would activate this old belief. Even if it wasn't true that we are lazy, our belief would convince us otherwise. We will be besieged and flooded with evidence that we are, in fact, lazy. We march to this beat and sit at its feet. Without realizing, we have given up our soul to it.

Imagine growing up hating people of color because our parents taught us the belief that they are inferior and evil. Our mental real estate is filled with words and imagery that support these claims.

Our parents fed us a PhD dissertation on reasons we need to adhere to this belief. By the time we can fully speak, we are a full-on follower of their racism.

Now, fast-forward thirty years. You are at a job and your boss is a person of color. Imagine your feelings and your inner resistance. This person is intelligent, compassionate, and kind. Imagine your inner conflict. You may not be able to function. Your internal dissonance may be so strong that you sabotage your performance or even leave your job. What a tragedy that would be, especially if you were about to get a fabulous raise and be promoted to a higher position because the boss believed in you, wouldn't it? In these unfortunate ways we come to see how our beliefs stand in the way of reality.

Arriving at Emptiness

The thing we don't realize about our beliefs is how they contaminate our perception of our world. We don't realize how much our experiences are colored by our mental projections and stories. If we did, we would be in shock. It's almost like we have been living but have not been alive. We have missed the entire circus. As long as we are attached to our beliefs, we are chained by them. They dictate our potential and the visions we manifest. We simply cannot escape their limitations.

The Buddha believed that *nirvana*, or the state of final awakening, could only occur with the extinction of all beliefs. He taught that beliefs are false stories we conjure about life and ourselves that are a complete fiction and, therefore, filled with ignorance. Once we deconstruct our beliefs and release them, seeing them as false, we enter a state of "emptiness of mind." We can finally be free of their hold over us and live in the as-is of our reality as opposed to the as-if of our beliefs. We finally enter the present moment of our reality without the imposition of our past.

This entrance into reality as it is versus how we believe it *should* be is the beginning of emotional liberation. Until we enter presence, which by definition can only be entered without the projection of our mental stories, we will never truly live and instead will just constantly be in a state of enslaved reactivity to our environment.

The reclamation of our soul involves a demolishment of our inner attachments. It's like opening our closet and throwing out all our clothes and starting fresh. The empty closet may seem desolate at first, and this can scare us, or it could feel like a blank space in which endless possibilities exist. This is what *emptiness* means in spiritual practice—entering a blank state whereby the present moment is experienced in its raw state without much contamination from our past.

To be empty is to enter a beginner's mind. Such a mind understands that to carry the past into the present is to be attached to the past. Through the emptying of our mind, we continually allow ourselves to enter each moment over and over again. Life is lived through the here and now as it appears before us. As such, we infuse the present moment with spontaneity and originality.

The Ultimate Law of Cause and Effect

When we live in the moment, we notice something profound. We pay attention to the chain of causes and effects in which we participate. We see how things came to be. Because our awareness is keen and sharp, uncontaminated by stories from culture, we can pay close attention to the causes and effects of life. We see how every effect came through a cause that was the effect of another cause before that. We see our influence in all these causes and effects. Everything is continuously in a state of becoming. Nothing ever is fully in a final state. As such, everything is in process. Nothing is ever at its final destination.

We now arrive at the profound realization that there is no beginning or end. Everything is constantly becoming, with more becoming, and then more. Everything rises and falls through interdependent origination. Life is an endless stream of causes and effects, rising and falling constantly. Therefore, nothing has intrinsic value or significance on its own. Everything is an amalgamation of causes and effects. Death and destruction are an inextricable part of this. Everything is essentially "empty" of its own value. This is what the concept of "emptiness" means.

We soon realize that this "I" that we label our "self" isn't a fixed "I," but an ever-fluid, ever-changing state of energy that constantly shifts in form, direction, shape, and purpose. The self is not an entity that we can say, Aha, here it is! The moment we do this, it shifts into the next constellation of causes and effects. The "I" or the self is essentially "empty."

Understanding the impermanent and interdependent nature of ourselves allows us to release our attachment to ourselves. We stop being obsessed with how we present ourselves to others or how others perceive us. We lean into the reality that we are never static but always dynamic and energetic, constantly shapeshifting. Once we realize this, we achieve a truer and deeper understanding of the concept of emptiness.

Once we understand the law of cause and effect on a deep level, we realize that our misguided focus on "a creator" is just a childish defense against the wondrous complexities of universal law. We see how religions needed to create a largely anthropomorphic entity that is omniscient and omnipotent. This figure is a surrogate father. Our reliance on this external source of knowing keeps us cut off from our own. It is so much easier to ascribe a starting point and a cause of it all, so that we can create order in our minds. Now, there is a beginning, middle, and end to the story which is far more reassuring to us humans than the realization that we can never know the beginning or the end. Accepting this is just too darn scary!

Once we understand nonduality, we now stop looking at the world through duality and instead see reality as it is, for what it is—an interplay of causes and effects. Because we realize that it's complex, nuanced, and inextricably interwoven through eons of evolution, we realize we may never know how it all began. Instead

of seeing this with defeatism, we see this with wisdom and acceptance. We tolerate the not knowing. Instead of seeking answers we
can never have and concocting all sorts of gods and goddesses, we
simply stay in the unknown.

To rest in this space of groundlessness is to revel in the marvelous
mysteries of the universe. In fact, the more we pay homage to all that
we don't know, the more we pay homage to the infinite nature of
the universe. When we pretend to know how things began, we actually strip the universe of its wonder. To truly respect the mysterious
glory of this universe is to stay in the unknown.

There is no beginning or end. There is no "I" or "you." There is
only an ever-flowing interplay of interconnection and interdependence. The moment we can release ourselves from our attachment
to our form, we can surrender to the magic of our inner formless-
ness, our inner essence. We are mightily significant and hugely irrelevant all at once—something and nothing at the same time.

It's only when we can embrace this paradox of existence that we
set ourselves free. Once we do, we will finally see ourselves as we
truly are—an echo, a mirror, and an exact resonance of the cosmos
herself, as infinite as the vast galaxies—but at the same time as in-
finitesimal as a speck on a sunbeam.

When you arrive at your essential emptiness, you arrive at your
essence. This will mark the beginning and the continued becoming of your *radical awakening.*

Your transformation is now afoot.

Sister, you have arrived at the end of this book. What a journey
you have been on! You have deconstructed so much about yourself
and your world! Your family of origin, your many personas, your

cultural conditioning, and your biology. You may have been trig-gered at many points along the way and didn't want to continue on. Yet something kept you going. Something kept you turning these pages forward, and now, here you are.

You might be wondering, "Now what?" Your internal world has probably turned upside down and you may be wondering how all of this will integrate into your life. You may be overwhelmed. If you are, I am here to reassure you that this is just the beginning.

You have garnered many new insights along the way. Allow them to wash over you with their jewels of awareness. As you al-low these into your psyche, they will naturally move you toward new emotional spaces. Before you know it, you will begin to make new choices, and create new destinies for yourself.

You may not realize it just yet, but your entire way of thinking has been revolutionized. You now see things in a completely new way. This will cause you to shift toward new realities that resonate more with your new consciousness. Of course, this means you will release a lot of the old, including relationships. Trust that you can do this with compassion and love. Trust that you are deserving of the new.

The most profound shift I hope you will allow is that you will connect to yourself differently. That you will have your own back and trust your own voice. That you will see yourself for the magnif-icent being that you are and that you will put yourself first.

You are at the threshold of a new vision of yourself.
Lean in. Enter. You are ready.
Your new world awaits.

Index